ALLE ZEIT WACH
1842

# Shoulder Replacement

Edited by R. Kölbel, B. Helbig, and W. Blauth

Translated by T. C. Telger

With 94 Figures and 31 Tables

Springer-Verlag
Berlin Heidelberg New York
London Paris Tokyo

Professor Dr. R. Kölbel
Osterstraße 61, 2000 Hamburg 20, FRG

Oberarzt Dr. B. Helbig
Orthopädische Universitätsklinik
Klaus-Groth-Platz 4, 2300 Kiel, FRG

Professor Dr. med. W. Blauth
Orthopädische Universitätsklinik
Klaus-Groth-Platz 4, 2300 Kiel, FRG

German edition published 1987 under the title:
Schulterendoprothetik, herausgegeben von R. Kölbel, B. Helbig, and W. Blauth

ISBN-13:978-3-642-71627-0 e-ISBN-13:978-3-642-71625-6
DOI: 10.1007/978-3-642-71625-6

Library of Congress Cataloging-in-Publication Data.
Schulterendoprothetik. English. Shoulder replacement.
Translation of: Schulterendoprothetik. Includes index.
1. Artificial shoulder joints. 2. Shoulder joint-Surgery.
I. Kölbel, R. (Reinhard), 1937- II. Helbig, B. (Bodo) III. Blauth, W. (Walter), 1924-.
IV. Title. [DNLM: 1. Prothesis. 2. Shoulder-surgery. WE 810 S386].
RD557.5.S3813 1987 617'.5720592 87-4979
ISBN-13:978-3-642-71627-0 (U.S.)



2124/3020-543210

# Preface

This volume contains the proceedings of the Symposion on Shoulder Joint Replacement held at the Kieler Yacht Club in conjunction with the 35th Annual Meeting of the Northwest German Orthopaedic Surgeons at Kiel in 1985.

Since the advent of suitable implant materials hemiarthroplasty of the shoulder was explored in the 1950s; total shoulder joint replacement was first reported in 1971. As interest in solutions to problems of the shoulder is growing, it appeared timely to present to interested clinicians the possibilities and limitations of a procedure as seen after nearly two decades of trials and experience. This volume is meant to give a comprehensive overview of the bases, the development, the alternatives, the state of the art and an outlook on some future trends.

The number of patients with problems warranting shoulder arthroplasty is relatively small. We consider this a blessing. This may be the reason why the number of surgeons who ventured in this field has remained small, even after implants became available - testimony of an awareness, that shoulder surgery is difficult.

The editors consider themselves fortunate to have been able to call on a number of those individuals, who were involved in first trials and in their evaluation. The editors are especially indebted to those from overseas who took it upon themselves to come, share their experience and join in the discussion.

It will become apparent to those readers already familiar with the subject, that in this international concert of voices there is a "cantus firmus", a tribute to one of the pioneers, whose teachings have influenced many of us - Charles S. Neer II.

We make the following acknowledgements with gratitude:

To Springer-Verlag for excellence in cooperation and in the producing of this volume; to our congenial translator; to the outstanding team of conference interpreters at the symposion, Mrs. K. Band, Dr. A. Beisel and Mr. E. Feldweg and to the staff of the Department of Orthopaedic Surgery, University of Kiel, for their help in organizing the symposion.

Hamburg, 1987 The Editors

## List of Contributors


Bergmann, G., Dr.-Ing.
Freie Universität Berlin, Orthopädische Klinik (Oskar-Helene-Heim)
Biomechanik-Labor, Clayallee 229, D-1000 Berlin 33

Bousquet, G., Prof.
Centre Hospitalier Régional et Universitaire de St. Etienne, F-42023 Saint Etienne

Braatz, D., Dr. med.
Orthopädische Abteilung Rheumaklinik, D-2357 Bad Bramstedt

Burri, C., Prof. Dr. med.
Abteilung für Unfallchirurgie, Hand-, Plastische und Wiederherstellungschirurgie, Universität Ulm, D-7900 Ulm

Cofield, R. H., M. D.
Mayo Medical School, Consultant in Orthopedic Surgery, Mayo Clinic, Rochester, Minnesota 55905, USA

Engelbrecht, E., Dr. med.
Endo-Klinik, Holstenstr. 2, D-2000 Hamburg 50

English, E., M. D., B. A., F. R. C. S. (C)
Orthopaedic Surgery Reconstructive Foot Care, Two Park Centre, 895 Don Mills Road, Suite 108, Don Mills, Ontario M3C 1W3, Canada

Gazielly, D., Dr.
Centre Hospitalier Régional et Universitaire de St. Etienne, F-42023 Saint Etienne

Heinert, D., Dr. med.
Endo-Klinik, Holstenstr. 2, D-2000 Hamburg 50

Jolles, C. W., Dr. med.
Orthopädische Universitätsklinik, Meibergdreef 9, NL-1105 Amsterdam-Zuidoost

Kölbel, R., Prof., Dr. med.
Osterstr. 61, D-2000 Hamburg 20

Knahr, K., Doz., Dr. med.
Orthopädisches Krankenhaus Wien-Gersthof, Wielemannsgasse 28, A-1180 Wien

Laumann U., Priv.-Doz. Dr. med.
Ltd. Arzt der Orthopädischen Abteilung, St.-Marien-Hospital, Am Boltenhof 7, D-4280 Borken/Westf.

Lettin, A., B.Sc., M.S., F.R.C.S.
St. Bartholomew's Hospital, The Middlesex Hospital and Royal National Orthopaedic Hospital, 45-51 Bolsover Street, GB-London W1P 8AQ

Lim, T.E., Dr. med., Oberarzt
Orthopädische Universitätsklinik, Meibergdreef 9, NL-1105 Amsterdam-Zuidoost

Marti, R., Prof. Dr. med., Direktor
Orthopädische Universitätsklinik, Meibergdreef 9, NL-1105 Amsterdam-Zuidoost

McElwain, J.P., M.B., F.R.C.S. (I), Tralee General Hospital, Kerry, Ireland

Pahle, J.A., M.D., Director
Orthopaedic Surgery, Oslo Sanitetsforening, Rheumatism Hospital, Akkersbakken N-27, Oslo 1

Raunio, P., Prof. Dr. med.
Rheumatism Foundation Hospital, SF-18120 Heinola 12

Rehder, U., Dr. med.
Universitätskrankenhaus Eppendorf, Orthopädische Klinik, Martinistr. 52, D-2000 Hamburg 20

Salzer, M., Prof. Dr. med.
Vorstand des Orthopädischen Krankenhauses Wien-Gersthof, Wielemannsgasse 28, A-1180 Wien

Salzer-Kuntschik, M., Prof., Dr. med.
Orthopädisches Krankenhaus Wien-Gersthof, Wielemannsgasse 28, A-1180 Wien

Sekera, J., Dr. med.
Orthopädische Krankenanstalt Wien-Gersthof, Wielemannsgasse 28, A-1180 Wien

Tillmann, K., Prof. Dr. med.
Leiter der Orthopädischen Abteilung, Rheumaklinik, D-2357 Bad Bramstedt

Watson, K.C., M.D.
1100 West Dannon, Fort Worth, Texas 76104, USA

Welsh, R.P., M.B., Ch.B., F.R.C.S. (C), F.A.C.S.
Orthopedic and Arthritis Hospital, University of Toronto, Toronto, Ontario, Canada

Wolff, R., Dr. med., Oberarzt
Orthopädische Klinik und Poliklinik der Freien Universität Berlin, Oskar-Helene-Heim, Clayallee 229, D-1000 Berlin 33

# Contents

# History

# The History of Shoulder Joint Replacement

R. Wolff and R. Kölbel

Prosthetic replacement of the shoulder joint is not utilized as freely or as frequently as in weight-bearing joints such as the hip. Arthrodesis and resection- or interposition-type arthro- plasties are still commonly performed today, although joint replacement is, in suitable cases, able to give more satisfying results in terms of pain relief, stability, and function.

The first artificial shoulder joint was implanted on March 11, 1893, by J. E. Pean (1830–1898) in Paris. When a 37-year-old man with a destructive tuberculous process of the upper humerus refused disarticulation, Pean implanted a constrained prosthesis made of hard rubber and platinum. Simple resection of the proximal humerus would not have given an acceptable result because of the extent of the osseous involvement. Pean considered ivory a poor prosthetic material because of its absorbability. The wound was closed with interrupted horsehair sutures, and a rubber tube was inserted for drainage. The patient made a good recovery and could walk about the ward 12 days after operation. However, a fistula developed postoperatively that did not respond to further measures, and the prosthesis was removed two years later.

The prosthesis (Fig. 1) consisted of a platinum stem and a hard rubber ball which was crossed by two deep grooves placed at right angles to each other. The grooves contained two platinum loops, one attached to the humerus and the other to the scapula.

Hard rubber is definitely unsuitable as an implant material, and the design of the Pean prosthesis casts serious doubts on its longevity. Nevertheless, an important first step had been made.

In 1914 the German surgeon F. König [23] replaced the upper end of the humerus with a prosthesis made of ivory.

Besides tuberculosis, the proximal humerus may be destroyed by neoplasia or by trauma. Replacement with an acrylic prosthesis (Fig. 2) [1, 11, 42, 47] proved unsatisfactory because of the poor functional result, and because the material and its anchorage could not guarantee long-term success.

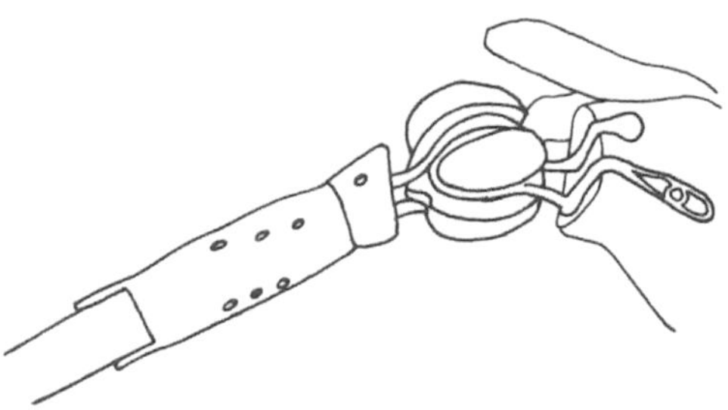

**Fig. 1.** Shoulder prosthesis of J. E. Pean [35]

Shoulder Replacement
Eds.: Kölbel/Helbig/Blauth

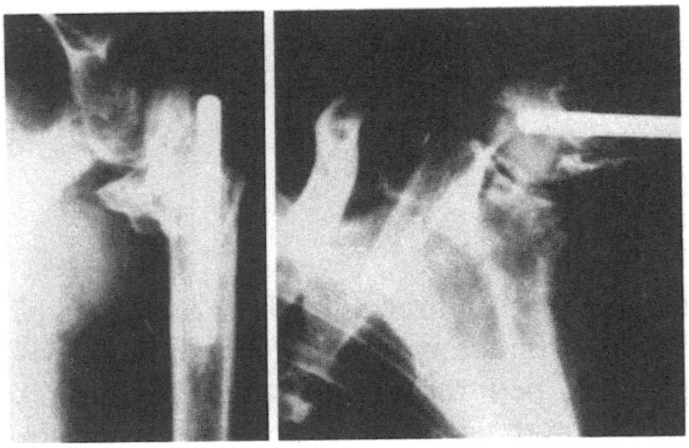

**Fig. 2.** Acrylic prosthesis of Judet [42]

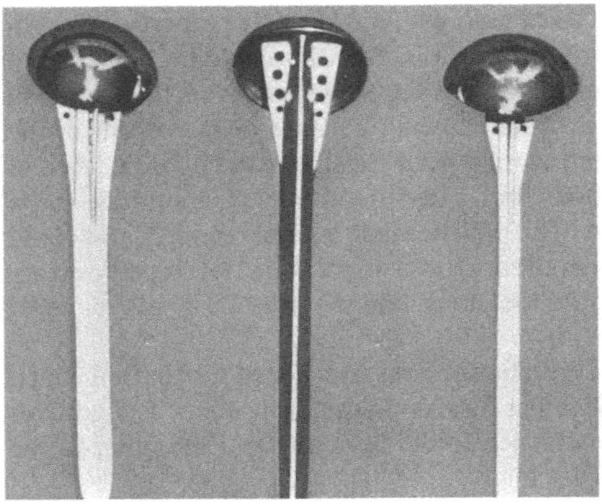

**Fig. 3.** Humeral head prosthesis of Neer [31]

In 1951 Krueger [24] described a Vitallium humeral head prosthesis whose stem was fenestrated to allow permeation by cancellous bone and improve the stability of the anchorage.

Venable [48] in 1952 designed a prosthesis for replacement of the proximal humerus. In 1953 De Anquin [7] published his experience with the prosthetic treatment of humeral head fractures (acrylic prosthesis in 1952, metal in 1956) [8].

Neer [30] was the first to report on humeral head replacements in a larger clinical series ($n = 12$). He first used his prosthesis for proximal humeral fractures and later broadened the indication to include degenerative diseases [31].

The articular surface of the Neer prosthesis (Fig. 3) reproduces the shape of the normal humeral head, except that it is flattened slightly on top to provide better seating in the area of the greater tuberosity and prevent impingement on the acromion. The original shape of the prosthesis was revised after the first implantations. Triangular fins in the cervical part of the device improve fixation and rotatory stability. A hole in the neck of the prosthesis can accommodate a wire for stabilizing the fragments of the greater tuberosity or for wiring bone fragments to the implant. The arthroplasty provided pain-free motion in 11 of the first 12 patients treated.

In 1964 Neer [31] reported on a series of 45 patients, noting that indications for the prosthesis were infrequent. He emphasized that degenerative diseases should be treated conservatively as long as possible, but that certain fracture dislocations of the shoulder justify primary treatment with a prosthesis, since the danger of later periarticular calcifications increases after three days. The prosthesis was further modified by placing perforations in the upper part of the stem for bone ingrowth (all the prostheses were implanted without cement!).

In Europe the polyacetal prosthesis of Mathys [28, 29] quickly found wide application for a variety of indications (fractures, tumors, rheumatoid arthritis). The humeral head prosthesis was designed in 1970 and later was supplemented by a polyethylene glenoid component attached with cement.

The prostheses come in a range of sizes so that they can be accurately matched to the humeral shaft. The implant has a slightly conical shape at the stem-shaft interface to strengthen the prosthesis and to improve stress transfer. The stem has recesses for bone ingrowth, with longitudinal grooves stabilizing the component against rotational forces and circular grooves against axial loads. There are holes in the proximal end of the prosthesis to allow reattachment of the rotators. A separate screw provides for primary rotatory stability. Burri et al. [6] rated the early results in a collective study (80 patients from 30 hospitals followed an average of 12 months) as fair, and in 1983 Burri [5] reported on a total of 166 implantations.

Until 1970 virtually all shoulder replacement arthroplasties involved replacement of the humeral head only (hemiarthroplasty), with the Neer prosthesis finding the widest application. While stem anchorage with these implants is usually very good, the success of the arthroplasty depends critically on the state of the shoulder muscles, most notably the rotator cuff, which keeps the head of the humerus centered in the glenoid cavity. If the glenoid is also involved by disease, its replacement should be considered as well.

This approach was first taken by Lettin and Scales [26] with the Stanmore total shoulder prosthesis, and later by Reeves et al. [41], Zippel [54], and Neer and Mathys, who supplemented their humeral head prostheses with glenoid components:

1969 Scales and Lettin (Stanmore)
1971 Reeves and Jobbins (Leeds)
1972 Zippel
1972 Kölbel
1973 Neer
1973 Post
1973 Kessel
1975 Engelbrecht and Stellbrink
1975 Beddow and Elloy (Liverpool).

These prostheses, which run the gamut from constrained to unconstrained designs, will be described below briefly in chronologic sequence.

When extensive damage occurs to the muscles that stabilize the shoulder and to important sensory receptors in the tendons and capsule, the forces acting on the joint become unphysiologic and complex, and a stable artificial joint will transmit tension, shear, and bending moments in addition to compression. This places stringent demands on the anchorage of the prosthesis - especially its attachment to the scapula. One difficulty is the relatively small amount of bone stock that is available in that region [21]. Thus, the attachment of the scapular component presents a special challenge, and the stability of the arthroplasty is limited by the quality of the anchorage of the implant to the bone.

All the prostheses described below have a ball and socket configuration in which a metallic head articulates against a polyethylene socket. A potential disadvantage of the ball and socket design, especially in constrained replacements, is that an impinging force becomes active during extreme limb movements. Moreover, tensile forces are transmitted by the prosthesis. Because this type of joint is used in shoulders in which the rotator cuff is destroyed, the resultant force vector assumes a more vertical orientation [49]. The methods of attachment of the glenoid component are variable, and some systems employ a reversed ball and socket configuration.

## The Stanmore Shoulder and Leeds Shoulder

The Stanmore shoulder (Fig. 4) has a humeral component that resembles the femoral component of an artificial hip. It is anchored in the humerus with cement. The glenoid component - also made of cobalt-chromium alloy - has anchoring posts for attachment in the glenoid cavity. The glenoid fossa and scapular neck are deepened by removing the cancellous bone with a curet. The center of the joint is displaced medially, which may affect the efficiency of the deltoid. (This alone cannot account for the poor range of motion of this arthroplasty.)

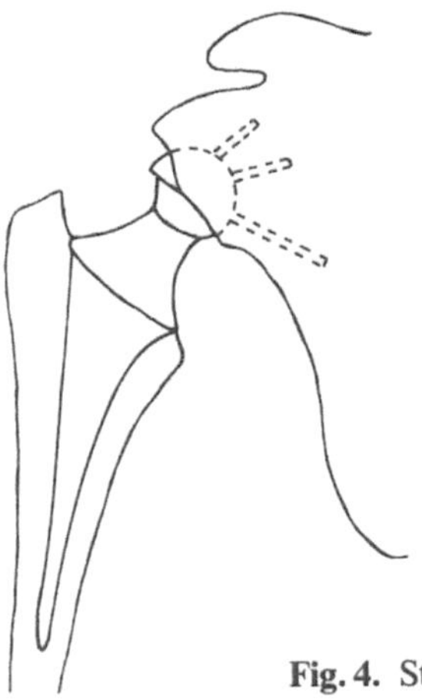

**Fig. 4.** Stanmore shoulder of Lettin and Scales (manufactured since 1969)

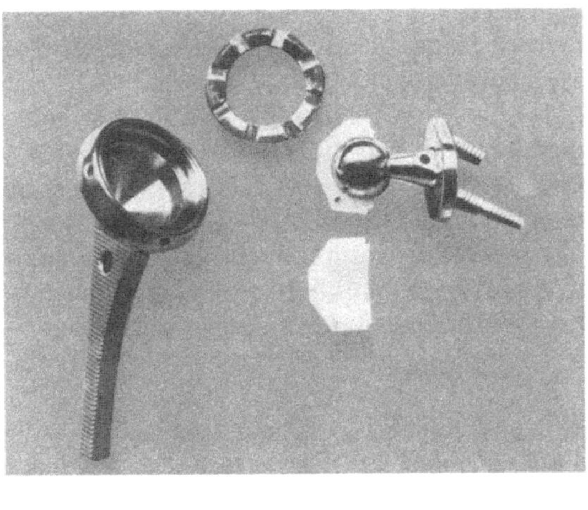

**Fig. 5.** Leeds Shoulder of Reeves et al. [41]

In the constrained Leeds shoulder of Reeves et al. [41] (Fig. 5), the center of the artificial joint coincides with the anatomic center. The instant motion center of the Stanmore shoulder is constant, and this is consistent with the mechanics of the normal human shoulder as characterized by Poppen and Walker [36]. According to Wallace [50], however, it is more likely that the humeral head normally makes an upward and downward excursion in the glenoid cavity when the arm is elevated and lowered (up to 10 mm in patients under 30 years old). Moreover, abduction of the arm is associated with an automatic external rotation, which is neglected in many total implants, especially the constrained types, and which may be one reason for their disappointing function [50].

As the Stanmore total shoulder evolved it acquired a semiconstrained design by the addition of an inner plastic ring to the glenoid component; also the humeral stem was shortened slightly [27]. The results of 50 arthroplasties performed between 1969 and 1977 have been critically reviewed [25, 27]. Nine prostheses had to be removed, and the loosening rate of the glenoid unit was relatively high. The latter was due in part to the small amount of bone stock available in the scapula. Excavation of the subglenoid bone often leaves behind an exophytic rim that does not allow for a stable prosthetic anchorage.

Zippel [51-54] in 1970 developed a dislocation-proof prosthesis with a fixed fulcrum. A retaining ring holds the metal head securely in the polyethylene cup. The dimensions of the prosthesis are small so that one model will fit all patients, and to minimize the size of the implanted foreign material. The range of motion of a ball and socket joint depends on the ratio of the head and neck diameters up to the point of impingement. A neck diameter of 4.5 mm was considered sufficient, while the head diameter (here 30 mm) cannot be increased arbitrarily for anatomic reasons. Zippel rated his early results in 11 patients as good [54], but 4 prosthetic neck fractures occurred in arthroplasties done elsewhere. For this reason the neck diameter was increased by 1 mm, although Zippel still considers the neck to be the weak point of the system. Insertion of the glenoid unit, which is attached with cement and two screws, requires some preliminary reaming of the glenoid cavity, which presumably increases the danger of loosening. Today this model is no longer used.

The Kolbel prosthesis [19-22] employs two means of protecting the attachment to the scapula. First, it limits the transfer of potentially damaging torques to the implant by allowing the joint to dislocate when a specific torque value is exceeded (here 9 Nm = newton meters); second, it extends the base of the fixation to cortical bone structures. This eliminates the effects of peak torques on the anchorage and reduces the stresses that accompany each load. The scapular component carries the ball and neck on a post which cements into the glenoid. A forked outrigger apposes to both aspects of the scapular spine and is clamped tightly against the bone with a transfixing screw placed through a drill hole in the cortical bone at the base of the spine. The humeral component is made of polyethylene and is cemented into the humeral shaft. The head of the prosthesis is secured with a retaining ring (Fig. 6). The joint has a 90° range of motion and permits rotation of the humerus about its long axis. Today the prosthesis is used only with modifications to reconstruct shoulders with tissue defects [19].

Neer in 1972 designed three types of fixed-fulcrum prosthesis that gave disappointing results. In 1973 he began using an unconstrained prosthesis with a polyethylene glenoid component, which was slightly modified in later years to improve its attachment. Neer listed the following requirements for a shoulder implant:

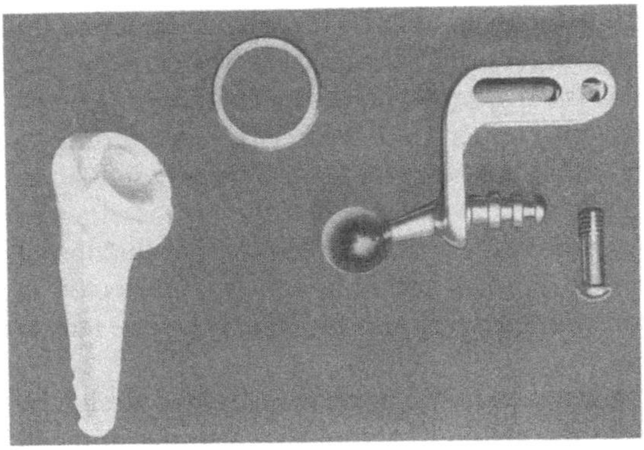

**Fig. 6.** Shoulder prosthesis of Kölbel and Friedebold [21]

1) anatomic shape for maximum range of motion;
2) minimum bone removal at insertion;
3) avoidance of mechanical blocking or impingement;
4) *repair and rehabilitation of the soft tissues* (rotator cuff).

In special situations a "semiconstrained" design is used in which the socket has a rooflike extension to prevent upward displacement of the humeral head.

The stem of the humeral component is fluted and usually is attached with cement. A series of 273 Neer total shoulder replacements (261 unconstrained) were performed from 1973 to 1981. In more than 75% of these operations the results were rated good or excellent [34]. Neer emphasizes the importance of meticulous repair of the soft tissues (rotator cuff) to minimize unphysiologic loads (shear) on the glenoid component. "It is the careful soft-tissue reconstruction which is the key to successful total shoulder replacement, not the device itself" [32]. Neer [33] reported on 500 consecutive shoulder replacements in 1984.

Kessel [2, 18] deliberately avoids fixation of the scapular component with cement. The metal ball (15 mm diameter) of his prosthesis, in use since 1973, carries a threaded post that screws into the glenoid cavity without cement. The polyethylene stem carries the socket, into which the ball is snapped. The stem is cemented into the humeral shaft. The center of the joint is displaced distally; this increases the distance between the acromion and proximal humerus and places the deltapectoral muscles slightly on stretch, increasing their efficiency [9]. Thirty-six shoulder replacements followed from 6 months to 7 years had an 80% "good" rating in terms of pain relief and function.

Post first implanted his constrained prosthesis in 1973, and he has used an improved version since 1976 [37-40]. The head and stem are made of metal (humeral component), and the head articulates against a polyethylene socket with an appropriate cavity. The diameter of the peripheral lip of the socket is slightly smaller than that of the humeral ball. The socket fits within a metal cup of truncated conical shape, which attaches to the scapula with a metal post. The metal cup and post are secured with cement and with two screws (also anchored in cement). A retaining ring holds the ball in the cup and allows dislocation of the prosthesis when a certain torque is exceeded. Initially the head diameter was 15 mm and that of the neck, 4 mm. Because of material failures (bending or breaking, see Zippel prosthesis), the components of Series II were made of cobalt-chromium alloy starting in 1976, and the humeral head and neck diameters were increased to 22 mm and 8 mm, respectively. Post emphasizes the importance of an intact glenoid (thus limiting the indications of the prosthesis!). The glenoid ordinarily contains enough cancellous bone for attachment of the metal glenoid component. The subchondral plate under the glenoid, where the trabeculae are most dense, and the underlying trabecular bone must be preserved. The trabeculae act as shock absorbers and permit a uniform dispersion of cement in the bone.

Twenty-four of the Series I prostheses were inserted from 1973 to 1975, and 11 of these required revision (dislocation, fracture of the neck, bending of the neck by trauma). From 1976 to 1982, 78 Series II replacements were performed in 74 patients (aged 31-80 years). Overall, the results were rated good in 73%, fair in 18%, and poor in 9%. Radiographs after 2 years showed radiolucent lines around the stem, screws, and anchoring post in 50% of cases.

In the Liverpool shoulder [4], in use since 1975, the head component resembles a hip prosthesis (Fig. 7). The stainless steel scapular component fits into the medullary cavity of the axillary border of the scapula (head diameter 20 mm). The grooved polyethylene socket is cemented into the proximal humeral shaft. Dislocation of the head is prevented by two diametrically opposed lugs on the cup extending just beyond the equator of the ball and reinforced by an external metal bracket. An initial prototype was designed in 1969. The reversed ball and socket design preserves the anatomic joint center and prevents impingement between the greater tuberosity and the acromion during abduction.

Of 19 prosthesis inserted, 16 were evaluated after periods up to 5 years. Good pain relief was obtained in 11 patients, and loosening of the scapular component occurred in 4 patients [4].

Other unconstrained prostheses have been described by O'Leary-Walker and by Engelbrecht and Stellbrink:

The St. Georg prosthesis was developed by Engelbrecht and Stellbrink [12, 13] from the Neer prosthesis and has been in use since 1971. The head and stem are made of chromium-cobalt alloy (head diameter 39 mm, stem length 105 mm). The standard polyethylene cup covers 1/4 of the head, and a model with a rooflike extension is available to prevent upward dislocation. Twenty-eight of these prostheses have been implanted since 1974 with good results [45, 12].

Other special prosthetic designs have been described by Fenlin [14], Swanson [46], Gristina [17] (trispherical prosthesis), and Grammont [16] (Acropole prosthesis).

Swanson [46] designed a kind of double cup prosthesis which completely fills the shoulder cavity, prevents impingement between the greater tuberosity and acromion, and allows the cup to align itself favorably in the glenoid. It requires no fixation of the glenoid component. Because motion occurs at two interfaces, the range of motion is potentially increased, and wear is reduced [46]. The prosthesis was developed in 1962 and used by the author in 15 shoulder replacements between 1976 and 1981, with good results.

In an attempt to increase the range of motion of a constrained prosthesis, Gristina [17] developed his trispherical total shoulder which combines two separate ball and socket articulations in one device. This design overlooks the fact that active movement under loading can take place only when one of the two articulations is in a position of impingement. The results of clinical trials were disappointing. A similar design was previously considered and rejected by Reeves et al. [41].

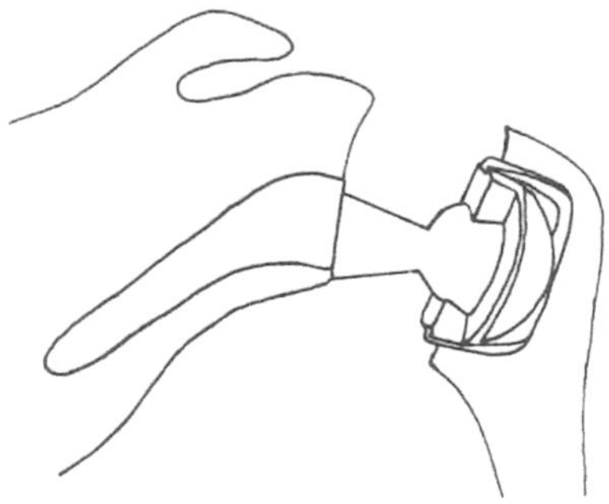

**Fig. 7.** Liverpool shoulder of Beddow and Elloy [3]

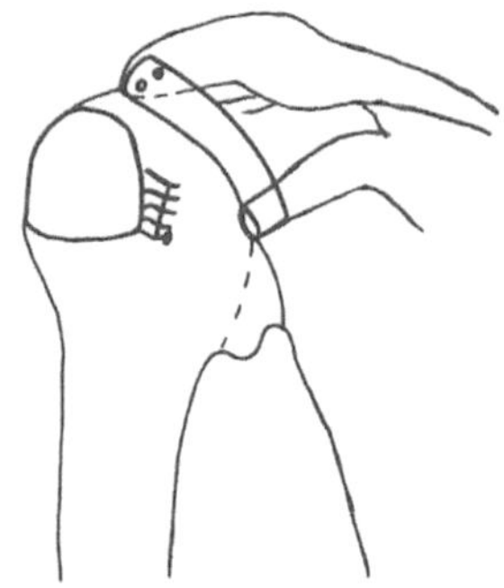

**Fig. 8.** Acropole prosthesis of Grammont [15]

The Acropole prosthesis of Grammont [15, 16] Fig. 8 employs a metallic, vault-shaped coracoacromial surface made of metal and fitted with 3 anchoring pins (1 for the coracoid and 2 others for the acromion, fixed with cement). The greater tuberosity is replaced with a polyethylene prosthesis which articulates with the metal gliding surface during abduction [15]. The prosthesis is used when it is necessary to resurface the subacromial articulation (e.g., for rheumatoid arthritis or severe, irreparable rotator cuff damage). The same principle was applied earlier by Clayton, who implanted a MacIntosh tibial plateau beneath the acromion to prevent upward displacement of the humeral head in patients with functionally deficient rotator cuffs (Gschwend 1976, personal communication).

## Outlook

The functional anatomy of the shoulder joint poses a unique challenge to prosthetic replacement. In many types of prosthesis, design deficiencies become apparent only after the device has been inserted and are based largely on an incomplete understanding of biomechanical relationships. Nevertheless, today we are able to identify with some accuracy the circumstances in which a partial or total shoulder replacement can provide a patient with lasting pain relief, function, and stability.

But function is not implanted along with the prosthesis, and integrity of the surrounding muscles is an essential prerequisite for a good functional outcome.

On the basis of biomechanical research, we may expect that further advances will be forthcoming concerning the reconstruction of large defects and the attachment of prosthetic components:

Salzer uses ceramic prostheses as spacers after proximal humeral resections for neoplastic disease (his article appears later in this volume). Rock et al. [43] of the Mayo Clinic obtained satisfying functional results with specially constructed titanium prostheses (module system), even after radical tumor operations (chondrosarcoma, osteosarcoma, fibrosarcoma).

Eckardt et al. [10], of the University of California, reported in 1985 at the annual meeting of the American Shoulder and Elbow Surgeons on 6 cases of scapular replacement with a fenestrated Vitallium prosthesis and a Dana polyethylene socket. Kölbel [19] reported in 1984 on partial scapular replacement with his modified prosthesis.

Through improvements in bone cement (carbon fiber reinforcement, bioactivation with apatite) and implantation techniques, shoulder replacement arthroplasty can be further optimized in older patients. Neer believes that it is unnecessary to experiment with cementless fixation, since to date he has not had to revise any of his cemented glenoid components [33]. He states that postoperative rehabilitation should not be hampered by an ingrowth-type component requiring special protective measures or immobilization.

The forces acting on the prosthesis and its anchorage also can be optimized by experiments with instrumented prostheses or by the use of computer models (finite element method) [44]. At present we know very little about the processes that occur at the implant-bone and cement-bone interface under functional conditions.

The first total shoulder implant was inserted by Pean in 1893. Sixty years passed before surgeons tried humeral head prostheses made of acrylic, and later of Vitallium, with the Neer prosthesis gaining a wide application that has continued, with modifications, to the present day. Concomitant resurfacing of the glenoid has been practiced since 1969. When there is significant functional deficiency of the rotator cuff, a constrained prosthesis is required. A number of prostheses with varying designs were developed in the early 1970s. Most are of the ball and socket type and differ chiefly in their method of attachment to the scapula. The models that have had the greatest clinical success will be described in the chapters that follow.

Today shoulder replacement arthroplasty has gained an established place in the treatment of shoulder disability. Expectant management, typified in Voltaire's remark that "the art of the good physician is to keep the patient's spirits high until nature cures him," can no longer be justified.

## References


1. Baron R, Sevin L (1951) Acrylic prosthesis for the shoulder. Presse Med 59: 1480
2. Bayley JIL, Kessel L (1982) The Kessel total shoulder replacement. In: Bayley J, Kessel L (eds) Shoulder surgery. Springer, Berlin Heidelberg New York
3. Beddow FH, Elloy MA (1982) Clinical experience with the Liverpool shoulder replacement. In: Bayley J, Kessel L (eds) Shoulder surgery. Springer, Berlin Heidelberg New York
4. Blauth W, Donner K (1979) Zur Geschichte der Arthroplastik. Z Orthop 117: 997
5. Burri C (1983) Isoelastische Schulterprothesen bei posttraumatischen Zuständen. Hefte Unfallheilkd 170
6. Burri C, Rüter A, Spier W (1977) Isoelastische Prothesen des Schultergelenkes - Ergebnisse. In: Burri C, Rüter A (Hrsg) Aktuelle Probleme in Chirurgie und Orthopädie, Bd 1, Teil I. Huber, Bern
7. De Anquin CE (1953) Fracturas de la extremidad superios del humero. Symposium 2° Congreso Latinoamericano de Ortopedia y Traumatologia. Rio de Janeiro Sao Paulo
8. De Anquin CE, de Anquin CA (1982) Prosthetic replacement in the treatment of serious fractures of the proximal humerus. In: Bayley J, Kessel L (eds) Shoulder surgery. Springer, Berlin Heidelberg New York
9. De Palma AF (1983) Surgery of the shoulder. Lippincott, Philadelphia Mexico City New York St. Louis Sao Paulo Sydney
10. Eckardt J, Eilber F, Jinnah R (1985) Endoprosthetic replacement of the scapula and shoulder joint for malignant tumors of the scapula: A preliminary report. American Shoulder and Elbow Surgeons, Annual Meeting (im Druck)
11. Edelmann G (1951) Immediate therapy of complex fractures of the upper end of the humerus by means of acrylic prosthesis. Presse Med 59: 1777
12. Engelbrecht E (1984) Ten years of experience with unconstrained shoulder replacement.

In: Bateman JE, Welsh RP (eds) Surgery of the shoulder. Mosby, St. Louis Toronto London
13. Engelbrecht E, Stellbrink G (1975) Total shoulder replacement - design St. Georg. Preliminary report. Scand J Rheumatol [Suppl] 4/8
14. Fenlin JM jr (1975) Total glenohumeral joint replacement. Orthop Clin North Am 6: 565-583
15. Grammont PM (1984) The Acropole prosthesis. In: Bateman JE, Welsh RP (eds) Surgery of the shoulder. Mosby, St. Louis Toronto London
16. Grammont PM, Lelaurin G (1981) Die Scapula-Osteotomie und Acropole-Prothese. Orthopäde 10/3
17. Gristina AG, Webb C (1982) The trispherical total shoulder replacement. In: Bayley J, Kessel L (eds) Shoulder surgery. Springer, Berlin Heidelberg New York
18. Kessel L, Bayley J (1979) Prosthetic replacement of shoulder joint: Preliminary communication. J R Soc Med 72
19. Kölbel R (1984) Stabilization of shoulders with bone and muscle defects using joint replacement implants. In: Bateman JE, Welsh RP (eds) Surgery of the shoulder. Mosby, St. Louis Toronto London
20. Kölbel R, Boenick U (1974) Biomechanische Probleme der Implantatchirurgie. Orthopäde 3: 153-163
21. Kölbel R, Friedebold G (1972) Möglichkeiten der Alloarthroplastik an der Schulter. Arch Orthop Unfallchir 76: 31-39
22. Kölbel R, Friedebold G (1975) Schultergelenksersatz. Z Orthop 113: 452-454
23. König F (1914) Über die Implantation von Elfenbein zum Ersatz von Knochen und Gelenkenden. Bruns Beitr Klin Chir 85: 613
24. Krueger FJ (1951) A vitallium replica arthroplasty on shoulder: A case report of aseptic necrosis of the proximal end of the humerus. Surgery 30: 1005
25. Lettin A (1982) Taking stock - ten years experience of shoulder arthroplasty. In: Bayley J, Kessel L (eds) Shoulder surgery. Springer, Berlin Heidelberg New York
26. Lettin AW, Scales JT (1972) Total replacement of the shoulder joint. Proc R Soc Med 65: 373
27. Lettin AWF, Copeland SA, Scales JT (1982) The Stanmore total shoulder replacement. J Bone Joint Surg [Br] 64: 1
28. Mathys R (1973) Stand der Verwendung von Kunststoffen für künstliche Gelenke. Aktuel Traumatol 3: 253
29. Mathys R, Mathys R jun (1977) Isoelastische Prothesen des Schultergelenkes. Werkstoffe - Instrumentarium - Prothesenmodelle. In: Burri C, Rüter A (Hrsg) Aktuelle Probleme in Chirurgie und Orthopädie, Bd 1, Teil I. Huber, Bern
30. Neer CS II (1955) Articular replacement of the humeral head. J Bone Joint Surg [Am] 37: 215
31. Neer CS II (1964) Articular replacement for the humeral head. J Bone Joint Surg [Am] 46: 7
32. Neer CS II (1970) Displaced proximal humeral fractures. J Bone Joint Surg [Am] 52: 6
33. Neer CS II (1984) Unconstrained shoulder arthroplasty. In: Bateman JE, Welsh RP (eds) Surgery of the shoulder. Mosby, St. Louis Toronto London
34. Neer CS II, Watson KC, Stanton FJ (1982) Recent experience in total shoulder replacement. J Bone Joint Surg [Am] 64/3: 319-337
35. Péan JE (1894) Des moyens prosthetiques destinés a obtenir la reparation de parties osseuses. Graz Hôp Paris 67: 291 (Nachdruck in: Clin Orthop 94)
36. Poppen NK, Walker PS (1976) Normal and abnormal motion of the shoulder. J Bone Joint Surg [Am] 58: 195-201
37. Post M (1978) The shoulder. Lea & Febiger, Philadelphia
38. Post MD, Jablon M (1983) Constrained total shoulder arthroplasty. Long-term follow-up observations. Clin Orthop 173: 109-116
39. Post M, Jablon M, Miller H, Singh M (1979) Constrained total shoulder replacement. A critical review. Clin Orthop 144: 135-149
40. Post M, Haskell SS, Jablon M (1980) Total shoulder replacement with a constrained prosthesis. J Bone Joint Surg [Am] 62/3: 327-335
41. Reeves B, Jobbins B, Dowson D, Wright W (1971) The development of a total shoulder joint endoprosthesis. Conference on Human Locomotor Engineering, Sept 1971. Institution of Mechanical Engineers, London, pp 108-122

42. Richard A, Judet R, Rene L (1952) Acrylic prosthetic construction of the upper end of the humerus for fracture luxations. Z Chir 68: 537
43. Rock MG, Franklin HS, Chao ES (1984) Limb salvage procedures for primary bone tumors of the shoulder region. In: Bateman JE, Welsh RP (eds) Surgery of the shoulder. Mosby, St. Louis Toronto London
44. Rohlmann A, Mößner U, Eberlein R, Bergmann G, Kölbel R (1983) Spannungsanalyse am Schulterblatt nach Schultergelenkersatz. Biomed Tech (Berlin) 28: 224-234
45. Siegel A, Engelbrecht E (1977) Schultergelenkendoprothese „St. Georg". In: Burri C, Rüter A (Hrsg) Aktuelle Probleme in Chirurgie und Orthopädie, Bd 1, Teil I. Huber, Bern
46. Swanson AB (1984) Bipolar implant shoulder arthroplasty. In: Bateman JE, Welsh RP (eds) Surgery of the shoulder. Mosby, St. Louis Toronto London
47. Van der Ghinst M, Houssa P (1951) Acrylic prosthesis in fractures of the head of the humerus. Acta Chir Belg 50: 31
48. Venable CS (1952) Shoulder prosthesis. Am J Surg 83: 271
49. Walker PS (1982) Some bioengineering considerations of prosthetic replacement for the glenohumeral joint. In: Inglis AE (ed) Symposium on Total Joint Replacement of the Upper Extremity. Mosby, St. Louis Toronto London
50. Wallace WA (1982) The dynamic study of shoulder movement. In: Bayley J, Kessel L (eds) Shoulder surgery. Springer, Berlin Heidelberg New York
51. Zippel J (1973) Arthroplastik des Schultergelenkes. Orthopäde 2: 107-109
52. Zippel J (1975) Der endoprothetische Ersatz des Schultergelenkes. Therapiewoche 28
53. Zippel J (1975) Luxationssichere Schulterendoprothese Modell BME. Orthop Praxis 11: 343
54. Zippel J (1977) Luxationssichere Schulterendoprothese Modell BME. In: Burri C, Rüter A (Hrsg) Aktuelle Probleme in Chirurgie und Orthopädie, Bd 1, Teil I. Huber, Bern

# Basic Principles

# Developmental History and Comparative Anatomy of the Shoulder

U. Rehder

## Ontogeny

The embryologic development of the human limbs becomes apparent in the fourth week of gestation, when paired limb buds sprout from the lateral aspect of the body, ventral to the somitic ridge.

Initially the limb buds are located in the cervical area just behind the origin of the hypoglossal nerve, and they are directed caudally, parallel to the trunk. With proximal growth they separate from the body wall and project at right angles to it.

As development proceeds, the entire limb bud becomes adducted toward the trunk. Subsequently the limbs undergo 90° of lateral rotation. This rotation brings preaxial muscle groups like the flexors, pronators, and adductors from a medial to a ventral position, and it brings postaxial muscles like the extensors and supinators from a lateral to a dorsal position. The caudal migration of the limbs commences in the second week of gestation.

Each limb bud, or epidermal protrusion, contains a mass of mesenchyme that is largely homogeneous initially. With further development the mesenchyme condenses, becomes concentrated centrally, and begins to form the future skeletal components of the arm and shoulder region.

The mesenchyme slowly becomes more compact and forms a precartilage which transforms into true cartilage as development progresses.

Ossification of the human skeleton begins at the center of the clavicle in the 5th-6th week of the embryonic period. Ossification of the humeral shaft and neck of the scapula begins in the 8th week. The humerus ossifies from 8 centers, as does the scapula. The clavicle has 4 ossification centers, 1 each at the ends and 2 coalescing in the diaphysis.

In the early stage of development of the joint capsule, the expansion of the scapular perichondrium onto the humerus serves as a capsule. It does not enclose the joint completely, however, and is absent anterosuperiorly.

The extracapsular ligaments appear quite early as zones of increased cellular density, examples being the coracoclavicular and coracoacromial ligaments in the 6th week.

## Phylogeny

Various theories exist on the phylogeny of the limbs, but so far none has been entirely convincing.

The *gill arch theory* of Gegenbaur (1865) rejects the independent formation of new skeletal parts in situ and states that the limbs developed from preexisting skeletal elements. According to this theory, the skeleton of the paired limbs is derived from the visceral arches. This means, for example, that the pectoral girdle (shoulder

Shoulder Replacement
Eds.: Kölbel/Helbig/Blauth

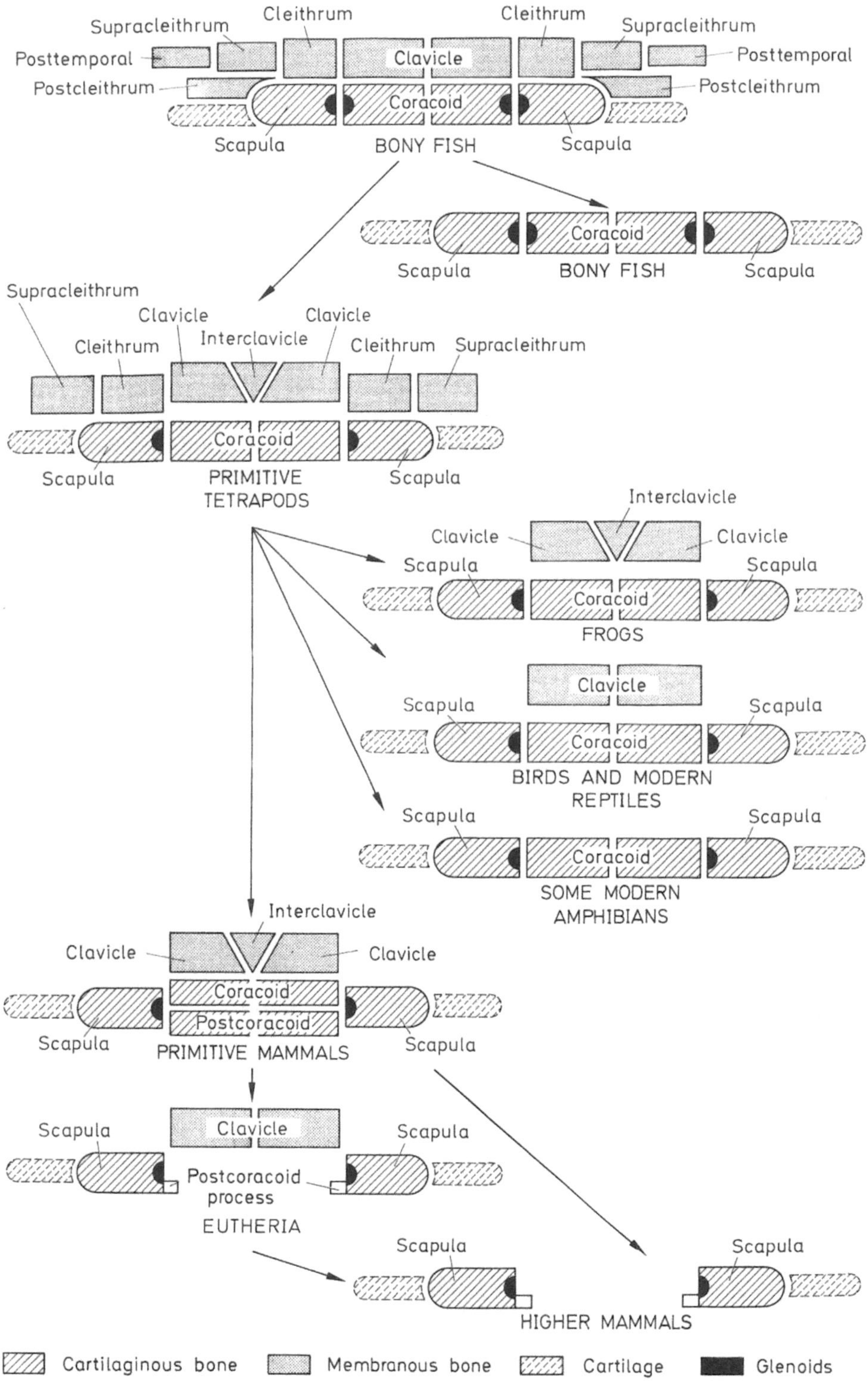
Supracleithrum
Cleithrum
Cleithrum
Supracleithrum
Posttemporal
Clavicle
Posttemporal
Postcleithrum
Coracoid
Postcleithrum
Scapula
BONY FISH
Scapula
Coracoid
Scapula
BONY FISH
Scapula
Supracleithrum
Clavicle
Clavicle
Cleithrum
Interclavicle
Cleithrum
Supracleithrum
Coracoid
Scapula
PRIMITIVE TETRAPODS
Scapula
Interclavicle
Clavicle
Clavicle
Scapula
Scapula
Coracoid
FROGS
Clavicle
Scapula
Scapula
Coracoid
BIRDS AND MODERN REPTILES
Scapula
Scapula
Coracoid
SOME MODERN AMPHIBIANS
Interclavicle
Clavicle
Clavicle
Coracoid
Postcoracoid
Scapula
PRIMITIVE MAMMALS
Scapula
Clavicle
Scapula
Scapula
Postcoracoid process
EUTHERIA
Scapula
Scapula
HIGHER MAMMALS
Cartilaginous bone
Membranous bone
Cartilage
Glenoids

girdle) and pelvic girdle each corresponds to a visceral arch. It is suggested that the actual skeleton of the free limb is derived from gill rays.

Objections that have been raised to the gill arch theory are that it does not account for the strong caudal migration of the pelvic girdle, and that the muscles of the limbs are of somatic rather than visceral origin. The latter claim is supported by their spinal innervation.

Moreover, ontogenic and paleontologic findings indicate that the primary position of the limb buds would have to be horizontal and not vertical if we were to assume that the limbs were derived from gill arches.

Another theory on the phylogeny of the limb skeleton, and one adopted by many authors, is the *lateral fin theory*. This theory stands in sharp contrast to the gill arch hypotheses by placing emphasis on the in situ development of the skeleton of the free appendages, independent of other skeletal members. It asserts that the primitive girdle was formed by an inward, peripheral-to-central extension of skeletal growth into the body wall from the free limb.

Neither of these theories can adequately account for all observations, however.

The evolution of the pectoral girdle is marked by the appearance and alteration of two skeletal elements. Just like the skull, the pectoral girdle contains two kinds of bones derived from desmal and from chondral ossification (Fig. 1).

The membranous bones derived from the skin progressively disappear during the course of evolution as the mobility of the organism increases.

The only membranous bone that has been retained in mammals is the clavicle. But it, too, has been lost in ungulates and whales, among others.

The situation is quite different with the cartilaginous bones of the pectoral girdle. The dorsal part, the scapula, and the ventral part, the coracoid, are very persistent over the course of the evolution. They disappear completely only when the entire forelimb is lost, as in snakes.

It should be noted that the coracoid of mammals is not homologous with that of amphibians, reptiles, and birds. For this reason it is commonly referred to as the postcoracoid in mammals. The coracoid and postcoracoid coexist only in the lowest order of mammals, the monotremes.

The limbs of the primitive reptiles are carried in a strongly abducted position, placing very heavy loads on the pectoral girdle (Fig. 2). The dorsal part of the girdle ossifies to form the scapula, which still lacks a spine and acromion. The ventral plate ossifies to form the coracoid.

The change in the mode of locomotion is accompanied by a change in the structure of the pectoral girdle. The predominantly bipedal locomotion of the herbiverous saurians leads to a complete regression of the membranous girdle. The clavicle

◄

**Fig. 1.** Evolution of the pectoral girdle (schematic), anterior aspect. (From Remane et al., Fischer-Verlag, Stuttgart 1976)

Key:

a. Posttemporal
b. Clavicle
c. BONY FISH
d. Interclavicle
e. PRIMITIVE TETRAPODS
f. FROGS
g. BIRDS AND MODERN REPTILES
h. SOME MODERN AMPHIBIANS
i. PRIMITIVE MAMMALS
j. Postcoracoid process
k. HIGHER MAMMALS
l. Cartilaginous bone
m. Membranous bone
n. Cartilage
o. Glenoids

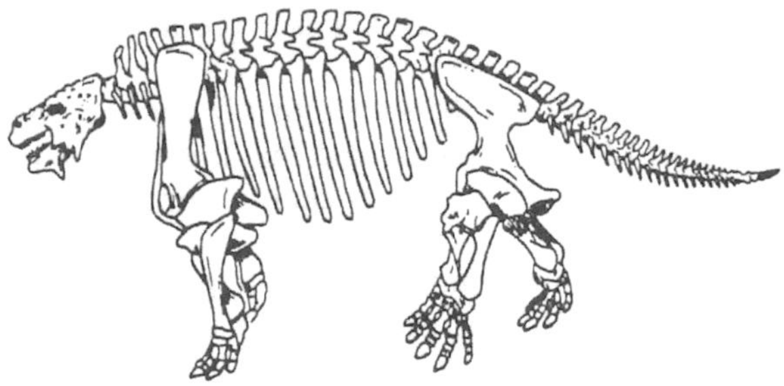

**Fig. 2.** Skeletal restoration of scutosaurus. (From Kuhn- Schnyder and Rieber, Thieme-Verlag, Stuttgart 1984)

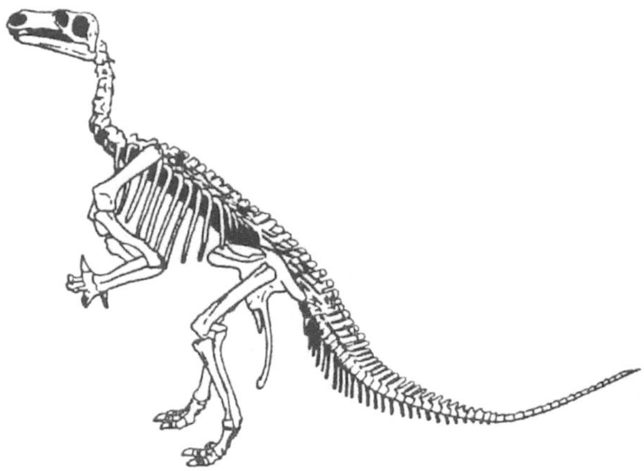

**Fig. 3.** Skeleton of iguanodon. (From Kuhn-Schnyder and Rieber, Thieme-Verlag, Stuttgart 1984)

and interclavicle are absent, and the procoracoid and scapula are fused. The scapula assumes an angled rather than a vertical orientation. The sternum does not ossify completely (Fig. 3).

The change to a swimming mode of locomotion also stimulates profound changes in the forelimb. The free forelimbs of ichthyosaurus, for example, become transformed into paddles. The humerus is greatly reduced in length. The pectoral girdle comprises a scapula, clavicle, interclavicle, coracoid, and sternum.

In birds, the acquisition of flight places new functional demands on the pectoral skeleton. The procoracoids become elongated and articulate against the strong, keeled sternum. The scapulae are relatively narrow and form a synarthrotic connection with the procoracoids. The furcula corresponds to the clavicles (Fig. 4).

In monotremes one finds an intermediate form between the reptilian and mammalian pectoral girdle. These animals have two large coracoids - the procoracoid and metacoracoid. In addition there is an interclavicle, a membranous bone of desmal origin.

Mammals exhibit an entirely new structural design of the pectoral girdle, consistent with their new mode of locomotion. The mammalian limbs are turned closer in to the body, so that the trunk no longer sags between the limbs as in reptiles but rests atop the limbs and is carried well above the ground.

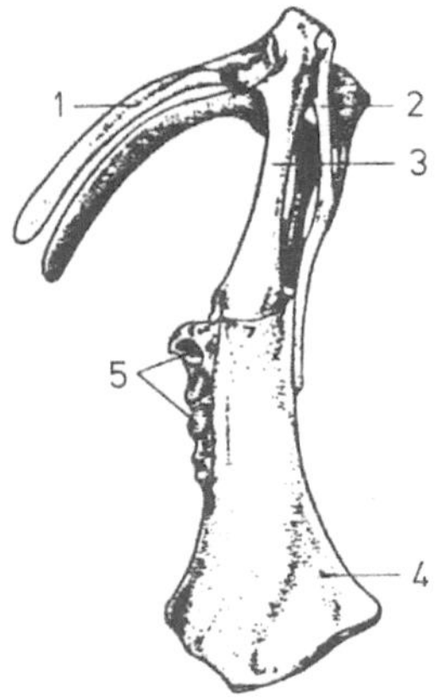


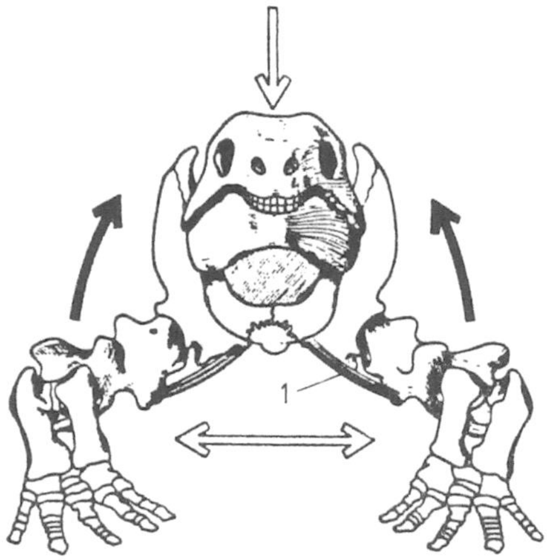


**Fig. 4.** **Fig. 5.**

**Fig. 4.** Sternum and thoracopectoral girdle of the hoatzin (Opisthocomus cristatus). 1 - Scapula, 2 - furcula, 3 - coracoid, 4 - crest of sternum, 5 - rib attachments. (From Starck, Springer-Verlag 1982)

**Fig. 5.** Diadectes (Cotylosauria), anterior view, showing the body load (vertical white arrow) and suspension of the pectoral girdle by the supracoracoideus muscle (1). (From Starck, Springer-Verlag 1982)

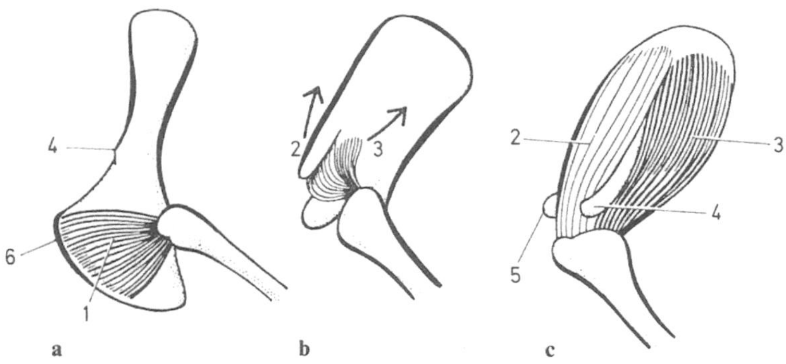


**Fig. 6a-c.** Changes in the structure of the shoulder region from the reptile to the mammal. **a** Lacerta, supracoracoideus muscle (1). **b** Didelphis (embryo). The supraspinatus (2) and infraspinatus (3) shift forward onto the scapula, as derivatives of the supracoracoideus. **c** Didelphis (adult). Acromion (4), coracoid process (5), coracoid (6). (From Starck, Springer-Verlag 1982)

In reptiles excessive sagging of the body is checked by a very powerful supracoracoid muscle, which arises from the coracoid plate and inserts on the humerus (Fig. 5). The mammalian posture eliminates the need for this arrangement, and accordingly we observe a phylogenic displacement of this muscle from the coracoid plate to the scapula.

This process can also be observed ontogenically in mammals, as for example in the development of the supra- and infraspinatus muscles in the opossum (Didelphis) (Fig. 6 a-c).

We see, then, that the two fossae are not equivalent formations. The infraspinous fossa corresponds to the old scapular plate, and the scapular spine corresponds to its anterior border.

The spine itself, like the supraspinous fossa, represents a new development in mammals, and we may interpret the bony plate forming the base of the supraspinous fossa as a muscular apophysis.

In the evolution of the pectoral girdle, this offers a rare example of Haeckel's theorem that "ontogeny is a recapitulation of phylogeny." Generally this hypothesis is not confirmed in observations of the embryology and paleozoology of the pectoral girdle.

## Summary

The phylogenic development of the pectoral girdle is characterized by a progressive decrease in the proportion of membranous bones comprising the girdle, while the cartilaginous bones are very persistent over the course of evolution.

It is obvious from comparative anatomy that the special structure of the forelimb is critically influenced by the mode of locomotion of the organism and thus by the nature of the functional demands that are placed on the extremity.

## References

Bolk L, Göppert E, Kallius E, Lubosch W (1938) Handbuch der vergleichenden Anatomie der Wirbeltiere, B 5. Urban & Schwarzenberg, Berlin Wien
Gardner E (1973) The early development of the shoulder joint in staged human embryos. Anat Rec 175: 503
Gardner E, Gray DJ (1953) Prenatal development of the human shoulder and acromioclavicular joints. Am J Anat 92: 219-276
Grassé PP (1967) Traité de Zoologie, Tome XVI. Masson, Paris
Kuhn-Schnyder E, Rieber H (1984) Paläozoologie. Thieme, Stuttgart New York
Lanz T v, Wachsmuth W (1959) Praktische Anatomie, Bd I, Teil 3 (Arm) Springer, Berlin Göttingen Heidelberg
Müntener M (1981) Funktionelle Anatomie des Schultergürtels. Helv Chir Acta 48: 523-532
Nelson OE (1953) Comparative embryology of the vertebrates. Blakiston, New York Toronto
Razek HA (1978) Atlas der Embryologie. Tabellenband. Enke, Stuttgart
Remane A, Storch V, Welsch U (1976) Systematische Zoologie. Stämme des Tierreichs. Fischer, Stuttgart
Romer AS (1971) Vergleichende Anatomie der Wirbeltiere. Parey, Hamburg
Starck D (1982) Vergleichende Anatomie der Wirbeltiere. Bd I-III. Springer, Berlin Heidelberg New York

# Kinesiology of the Shoulder Joint

U. Laumann

## Introduction

Kinesiology is the branch of biomechanics which deals with the description and analysis of movements in the *living* organism. In the shoulder-arm complex, it is concerned with translational and rotational movements of the clavicle, scapula, and humerus and studies the forces which are transmitted to this motor system by the numerous muscles around the shoulder.

In contrast to the lower extremity, in which movements are stored engrammatically and thus are reproducible to a high degree, movements of the upper extremity are always voluntary and purposeful and therefore are almost infinitely variable. To obtain comparable, reproducible results, it is necessary to have the upper arm move in constrained, designated directions, e.g., on the frontal and sagittal planes and on the plane bisecting these planes, called the scapular plane. To perform a spatial analysis of these movements, we need to have a three-dimensional recording system. We used stereophotogrammetry for our studies. Associated muscular activities were recorded by on-line computer electromyointegration.

## Results

## Position of Equilibrium of the Shoulder Girdle

The reference point and baseline for kinesiologic studies of the shoulder joint is the equilibrium position of the shoulder girdle in the resting posture. Because of the highly mobile muscular suspension of the shoulder girdle, whose only osseous connection with the axial skeleton is via the sternoclavicular joint, it is not possible to define a resting equilibrium position uniquely. This led us to investigate the resting position of the scapulae by stereophotogrammetry in a group of 40 healthy subjects, leading to the following results:

The resting position of the shoulder girdle varies as a function of posture, although it remains within definite limits.

In our study population the medial border of the scapula showed a mean cranial rotation ($\alpha$ angle) of 3° (±3°) and a mean anteflexion ($\beta$ angle) of minus 18.9° (± 10.0°); i.e., the inferior angle of the scapula deviates by this amount posteriorly from the frontal plane.

The mean inclination of the scapular spine anteriorly from the frontal plane ($\gamma$ angle) was 30.8°, and the mean distance from the medial end of the scapular spine to the vertical line of the spinal column (dist.) was 89.2 mm (see Figs. 1 and 2).

This equilibrium position is not maintained by active muscular effort; it is controlled entirely by the capsular and ligamentous attachments of the interposed joints and by the resting tone of the shoulder muscles. The major importance of the

Shoulder Replacement
Eds.: Kölbel/Helbig/Blauth

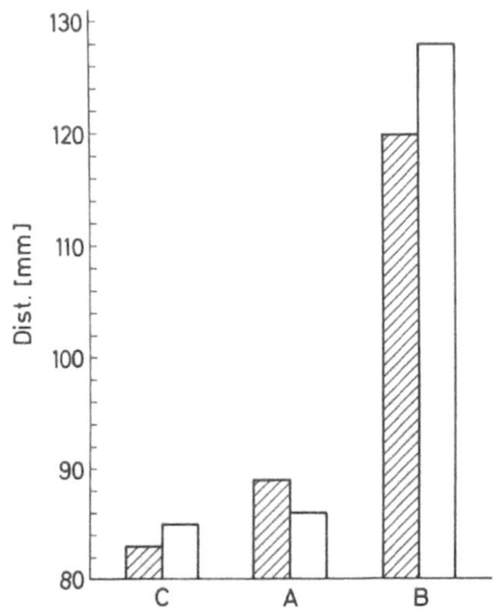


**Fig. 1.** Mean distance of the medial scapular spine from the vertical line through C7 (Dist.) with the arms at rest and with a weight suspended from the hanging arm (x = 8 kg in healthy individuals). A Healthy subjects, B trapezius paralysis, C serratus anterior paralysis, *filled columns* resting posture, *empty columns* weight

resting tone for physiologic equilibrium of the shoulder girdle is seen in the effects of trapezius or serratus anterior paralysis.

Isolated trapezius paralysis leads to an anterocaudal displacement of the shoulder girdle from the resting equilibrium position described above. In this situation loss of the posterior checkrein allows the shoulder girdle to be pulled downward by the intrinsic weight of the arm. As this occurs, the scapula becomes lateralized and turns in a parasagittal plane, and the coracoid process points downward. Meanwhile the clavicle moves progressively onto the frontal plane. With isolated paralysis of the serratus anterior, causing loss of the anterior checkrein of the shoulder, the direction of displacement is opposite to that in trapezius paralysis: the scapula becomes medialized and progressively turns onto a frontal plane, and the scapular distance is decreased (Fig. 1).

Under normal conditions, however, the equilibrium position of the shoulder girdle must be regarded as highly stable. We observed this in loading tests on the hanging arm with incremental weights of 1 to 20 kg. We found that even a 20 kg weight applied for 1 min did not cause the scapula to rotate significantly from the baseline position.

Concurrent electromyographic tests indicate that the shoulder girdle is kept in balance by appropriate tension from the pars descendens of the trapezius muscle and from the pars convergens of the serratus anterior. Closure of the glenohumeral joint surfaces is maintained by the muscles of the rotator tendon cuff, and not by the deltoid as one might expect.

## Dynamics of the Shoulder-Arm Complex

When muscular forces act on the shoulder-arm complex, the relatively stable equilibrium position of the shoulder girdle is lost: the humerus, scapula, and clavicle are accelerated and move relative to the trunk and to one another. We used the technique of stereophotogrammetry to follow the movements of the scapula during ele-

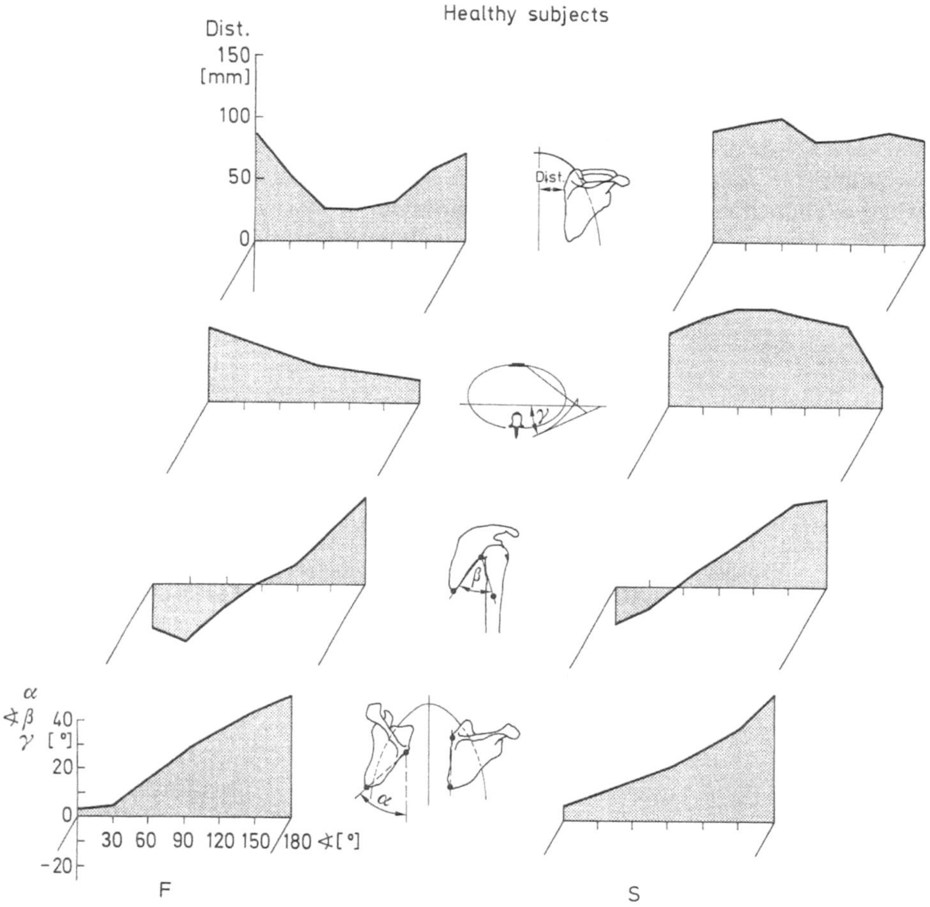


**Fig. 2.** Stereophotogrammetric determination of scapular rotation about the 3 spatial axes during arm elevation from 0°-180° on the frontal (F) and sagittal plane (S) (n = 40). $\alpha$ Scapular rotation projected onto the frontal plane, $\beta$ scapular rotation projected onto the sagittal plane, $\gamma$ scapular rotation projected onto the horizontal plane; Dist. distance between the vertical at C7 and the medial border of the scapular spine

vation of the arm on designated planes of motion, and we additionally used electromyography to record the muscular activities accompanying the movements.

Our findings: During the first 30° of arm elevation, the shoulder girdle moves from its resting equilibrium position onto the designated plane of motion. This process is not well ordered, as indicated by the marked variation in the direction of scapular rotation from one individual to the next. Our studies further indicate that this "setting phase" is much more pronounced and of longer duration during abduction of the arm than during anteflexion, or elevation on the sagittal plane. After the setting phase, the relationship between arm elevation and scapular rotation becomes linear and does not change with further abduction. During anteflexion of the arm a small degree of opposite terminal rotation is observed (Fig. 2).

The extent and direction of scapular rotation are determined by the plane of elevation of the arm. This is most apparent during the initial movement of the scapular spine ($\gamma$ angle), which on abduction moves toward the frontal plane, and on flexion rotates increasingly onto a parasagittal plane until terminal rotaton restores it to a more frontal orientation. These movements evoke translations of the scapula, as we see from the changing distance between the medial end of the scapular spine and the vertical line of the vertebral column (see Fig. 2). When the arm is raised to full elevation, the scapula always attains the same terminal position, regardless of whether abduction or anteflexion was performed.

When the arm is elevated, the inferior angle of the scapula moves laterally and anteriorly over the chest wall, a process that is evidenced by a change of sign

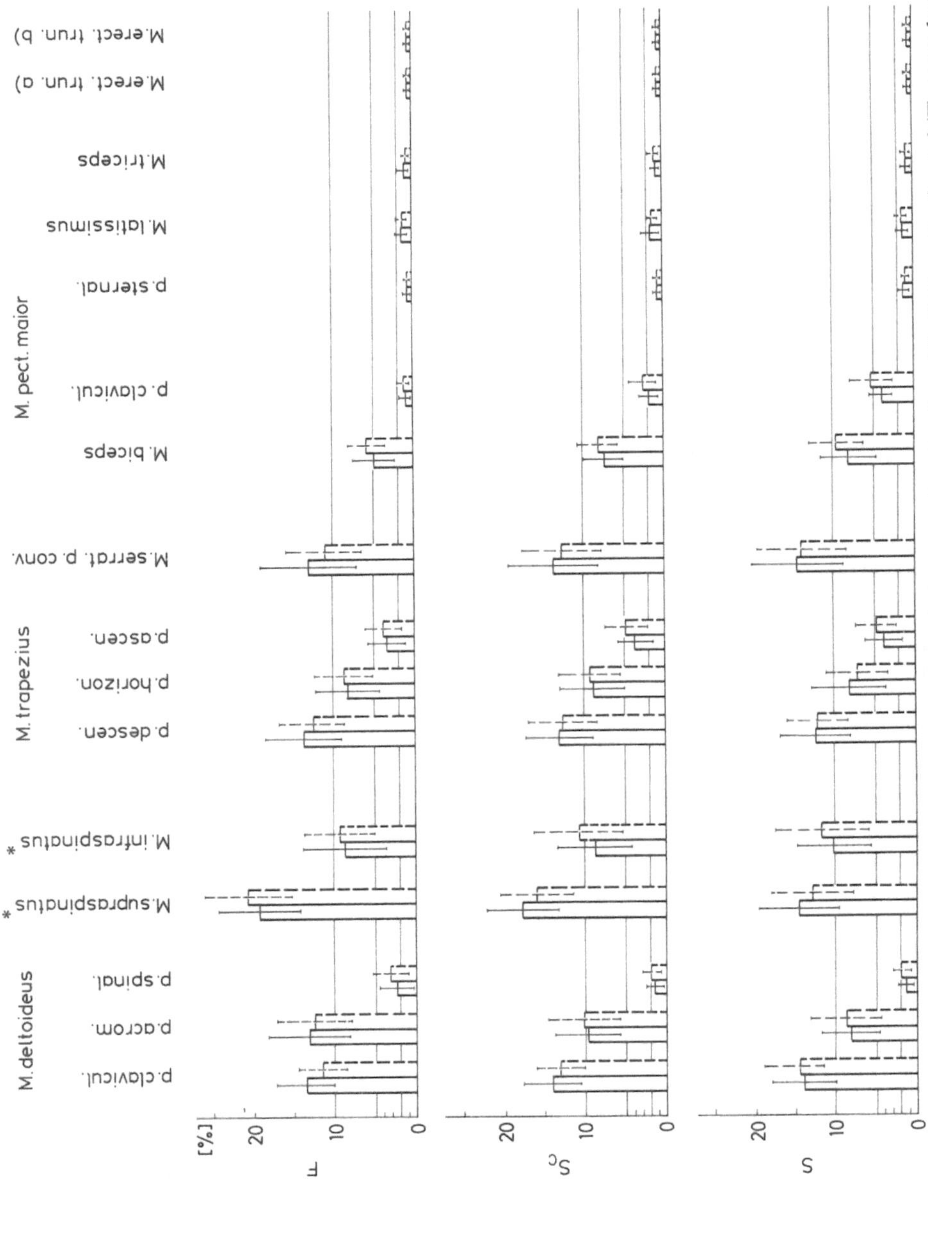


**Fig. 3.** Relative distribution of muscular activity during arm elevation from 0°–180° on the frontal (F), scapular (Sc), and sagittal planes (S). The *dashed columns* show the values with a counterforce of 30 N applied to the shoulder girdle

($\beta$ angle) on the graph. This is more apt to occur with anteflexion than with abduction.

The movements of the scapula are accompanied by synchronous movements of the clavicle about all three spatial axes, as Inman et al. have pointed out.

No fewer than 26 muscles act upon the shoulder-arm complex. When we tested the degree to which the various muscles participated in elevation of the arm, we identified only a few that made a significant contribution (Fig. 3).

We classified the muscles into four groups according to the relative distribution of muscular activities measurable during arm elevation. The muscles of group I are considered to be essential, as the loss of any one of them will cause a significant limitation of motion, which in some cases can be compensated by other muscles (Fig. 4).

Generally the loss of two essential muscles makes it impossible to elevate the arm appreciably. We have analyzed in some detail the activity patterns of the essential muscles and their coordinates during arm elevation (Fig. 5 a–d).

We found that a significant rise of activity was recorded from all of these muscles even at the start of the movement; this was particularly evident in the leads from the supraspinatus. Apparently the muscles of the rotator tendon cuff play a more important initiating role in moving the arm onto the prescribed plane of motion at the glenohumeral joint than do the clavicular and acromial parts of the deltoid.

Of the muscles acting on the scapula, the descending and horizontal parts of the trapezius muscle act more strongly on the shoulder girdle in this phase of movement than do the convergent fibers of the serratus anterior. After this "setting phase" and up to about 120° of elevation, there is a phase in which all essential muscles increase their activity in roughly linear fashion, except for the supraspinatus, which reaches its peak activity at about 60° of anteflexion and 90° of abduction. From 120° to 150° we observe a shift of muscular activities, with the clavicular and ac-

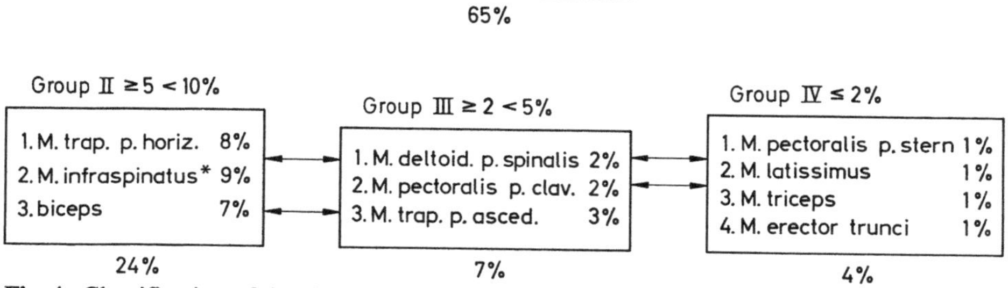


**Fig. 4.** Classification of the shoulder muscles into groups according to their total activity during arm elevation. Group I comprises the "essential" shoulder muscles (readings were not taken from the subscapularis)

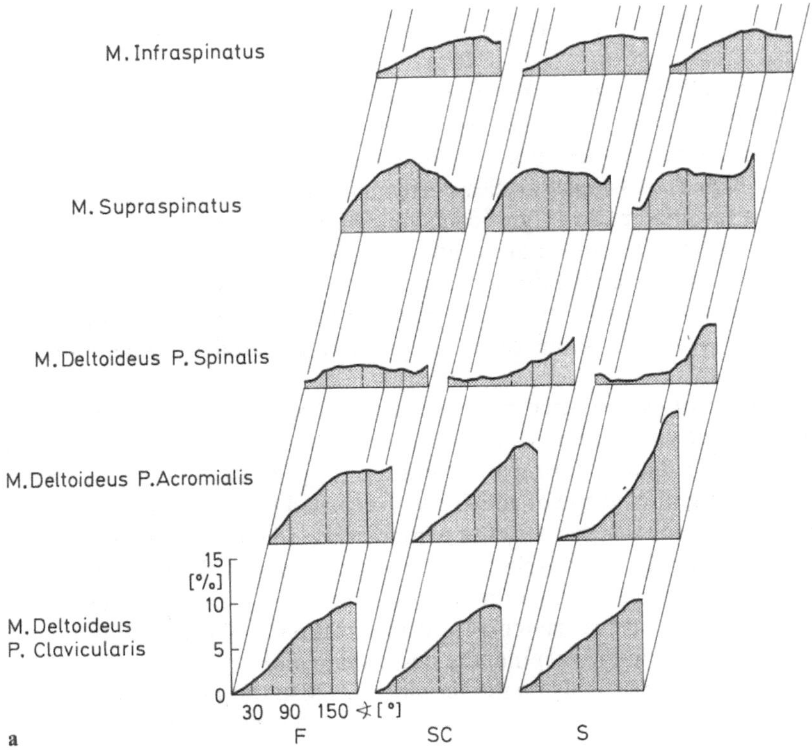


a

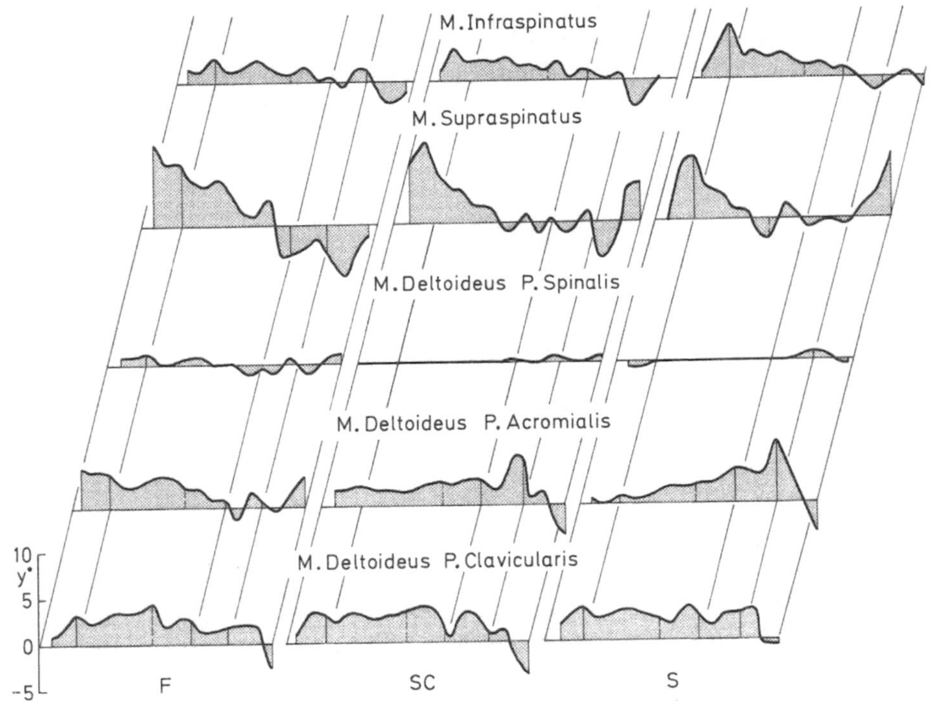


b

**Fig. 5. a,c** Patterns of muscular activity during arm elevation from 0°–180° for movements on the frontal (F), scapular (Sc), and sagittal planes (S); **a,d** show lead 1 ($\gamma$'), which reflects the pattern of rise of the curves

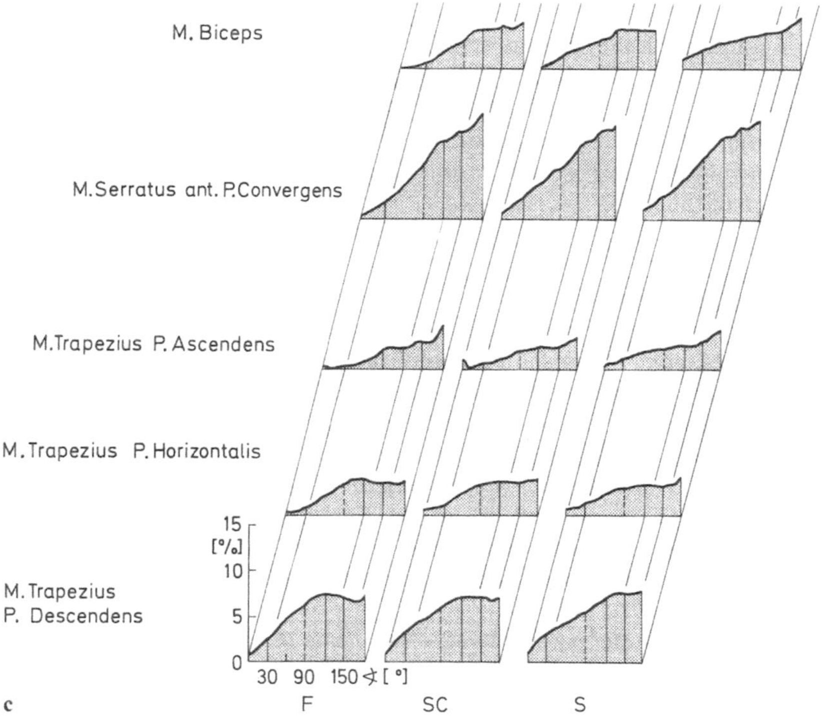
M. Biceps
M.Serratus ant. P.Convergens
M.Trapezius P. Ascendens
M.Trapezius P. Horizontalis
M.Trapezius
P. Descendens
15
[%]
10
5
0
30 90 150 ∢ [°]
F
SC
S

c

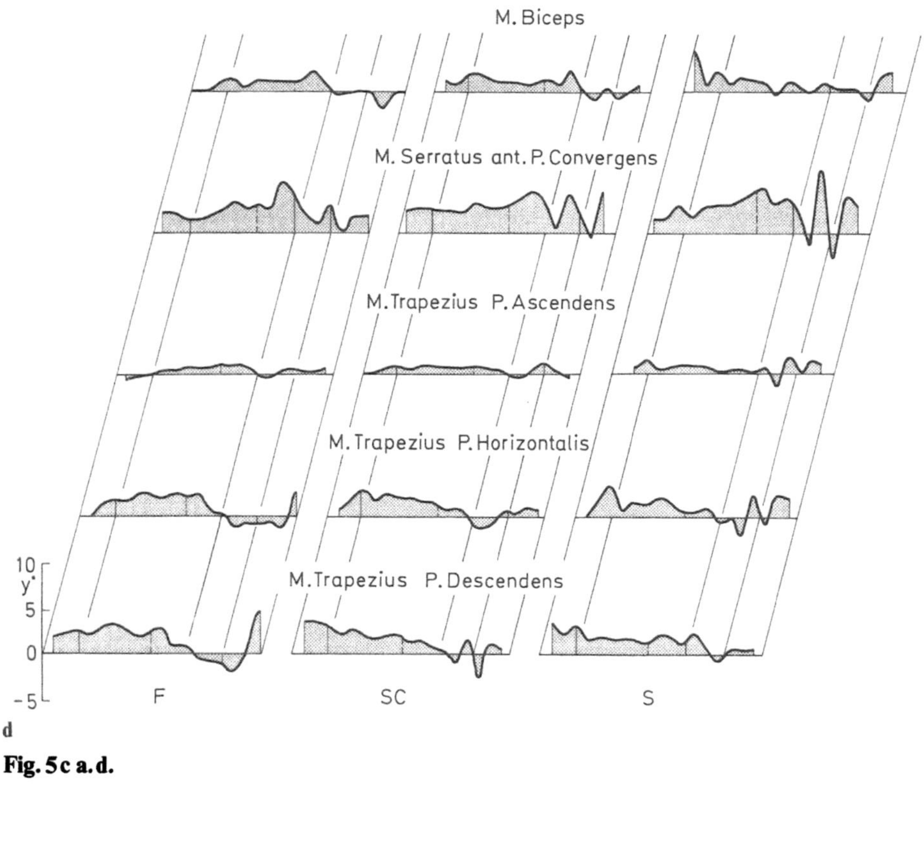
M. Biceps
M. Serratus ant. P. Convergens
M.Trapezius P. Ascendens
M.Trapezius P. Horizontalis
M.Trapezius P. Descendens
10
y''
5
0
-5
F
SC
S

d

**Fig. 5c a. d.**

romial parts of the deltoid becoming the principal motors of the humerus at the glenohumeral joint, while the serratus anterior becomes more active in continuing the movement of the shoulder girdle. In the final arc from 150° to 180°, regardless of the direction of arm motion, small activity peaks are registered over the acromial part of the deltoid, the supraspintaus, the descending and horizontal parts of trapezius, and the convergent fibers of serratus anterior. These activity peaks relate to the terminal rotation of the limb.

## Summary and Conclusions

Studies on the kinesiology of the shoulder joint show that the equilibrium position of the shoulder girdle is quite stable despite its mobile suspension. Movements in this complex system are initiated by the actions of a few "essential" muscles.

An initial *setting phase* that establishes the direction of arm motion is followed by synchronous *rotational* and *translational movements* of all the skeletal elements involved in the shoulder-arm complex. We can distinguish phases in the control of movement in which the suspensory muscles of one system act simultaneously and synergistically, from phases in which one component of the suspensory system increases its activity.

Accordingly, we may anticipate ordered movements of the shoulder-arm complex when the essential shoulder muscles are functionally intact, and the movements of the clavicle, scapula, and humerus can occur without hindrance at the associated joints. Thus, in order to make a prognostic assessment of shoulder function after total replacement arthroplasty, arthrodesis, or myoplastic reconstruction, we must first ascertain the state of the essential shoulder muscles, and we must test not just the functional status of the glenohumeral joint but also the functional status of the sternoclavicular (SC) joint, the acromioclavicular (AC) joint, and the scapulothoracic joint. A *total replacement arthroplasty* of the glenohumeral joint will be functionally unsound unless function has been restored to the muscles of the rotator cuff. An *arthrodesis* of the glenohumeral joint will not give a satisfying functional result when there is advanced degenerative disease of the AC joint that has not been concurrently treated by a resection arthroplasty.

By the same token, *myoplastic reconstructions* can improve function only when all lost essential muscles are reconstructed, e.g., when myoplastic replacement of the deltoid in C5 or C6 paralysis is supplemented by reconstruction of the muscles of the rotator cuff.

## References


1. Basmajian JV (1967) Muscles alive. Their functions revealed by electromyography. Williams & Wilkins, Baltimore
2. Bearn JG (1961) An electromyographic study of the trapezius, deltoid, pectoralis maior, biceps and triceps muscles during stating loading of the upper limb. Anat Rec 140: 103
3. Braune W, Fischer O (1888) Über den Anteil, den die einzelnen Gelenke des Schultergürtels an der Beweglichkeit des menschlichen Humerus haben. Hirzel, Leipzig
4. Brunnstrom S (1972) Clinical kinesiology. Davis, Philadelphia
5. Comtet JJ, Auffray Y (1970) Physiologie des muscles elevateurs de l' épaule. Rev Chir Orthop 56: 105
6. Dempster WT (1965) Mechanism of shoulder movement. Arch Phys Med Rehabil 46: 49

7. Fischer LP, Carret JP, Gronon GP, Dimnet J (1977) Etude cinématique des mouvements de l'articulation scapulo-humérale (articulatio humeri). Rev Chir Orthop [Suppl] 63/II: 108
8. Freedman L, Munro R (1966) Abduction of the arm in the scapular plane: Scapular and glenohumeral movements. J Bone Joint Surg [Am] 48: 1503
9. Hamonet C (1972) Étude electromyographique du muscle sus-épineux. In: Boitzy A, Müller ME (eds) Périarthrite de l'épaule, osteogenese et compression. Huber, Bern, 25
10. Inman VT, Saunders JB, Abbott L (1944) Observations on the function of the shoulder joint. J Bone Joint Surg 26: 1
11. Jonston TB (1937) Movements of the shoulder joint: A plea for the use of the plane of the scapula as a plane of reference for movements occuring at the humero-scapular joint. Br J Surg 25: 252
12. Latarjet M, Bouchet A (1963) Considérations sur le mouvement d'élévation du bras à la verticale. Bulletin de l'Association des Anatomistes II. Réun Eur Anatom 221
13. Laude M, Kénési C, Patte D, Riggs E (1978) Abduction and horizontal extension of the arm. Anat Clin 1: 65
14. Lucas DB (1973) Biomechanics of the shoulder joint. Arch Surg 107: 425
15. Moseley HF (1968) The clavicle: It's anatomy and function. Clin Orthop 58: 19
16. Poppen NK, Walker PS (1976) Normal and abnormal motion of the shoulder. J Bone Joint Surg [Am] 58: 195
17. Saha AK (1950) Mechanism of shoulder movements and a plea for the recognition of zero-position of the gleno-humeral joint. Indian Surg 12: 153
18. Saha AG (1961) Theory of shoulder mechanism: Descriptive and applied. Thomas, Springfield/Ill

# Biomechanics and Pathomechanics of the Shoulder Joint with Reference to Prosthetic Joint Replacement

G. Bergmann

The extremely large range of motion of the upper arm is made possible by the coordinated interaction of multiple joints, and the biomechanics of the glenohumeral joint can be studied and understood only in relation to the biomechanics of the shoulder as a whole. When the glenohumeral joint is replaced with a prosthesis, four closely interrelated problems arise that assume major importance:

1. *Contact of the joint surfaces* can be maintained either by the balance of imposed forces (unconstrained prosthesis) or by the geometry of the artificial joint (constrained prosthesis).
2. The possible *range of motion* of the joint depends on the selected design.
3. Both factors jointly determine the *loads* that are transmitted through the sites of attachment of the prosthesis.
4. The *loads on the bone* vary according to the manner in which the prosthesis is attached to the bone. These problems, together with the mechanical durability of the prosthesis and other factors, critically influence the long-term success of the arthroplasty.

If we consider the case of an arm that is moved through a full 180° of abduction (Fig. 1), we observe that only about half the motion (90°) takes place between the humerus and scapula. Relative motion also occurs between the scapula and clavicle and between the clavicle and sternum. The arm and hand acquire an additional action radius from the upright, freely mobile vertebral column. This articular arrangement, which is very unstable from a mechanical standpoint, is able to function because of the ingenious muscular suspension of the scapula, which gives the scapula a wide but stable range of motion on the chest wall.

The range of angular movement in the glenohumeral joint itself during vertical elevation of the arm varies from 60° to more than 120° according to reports by different authors (Fig. 2). However, simplified models of shoulder motion often neglect the fact that movements of the scapula and clavicle during abduction take place on more than just one plane, and so the above discrepancies may relate in part to the method used.

Different authors also disagree on the sequence of movements which occur during abduction of the arm (see Fig. 2). During an initial abduction of 30° (horizontal axis of the graph), curves 1, 2, 3, and 6 show that the whole of the movement takes place at the glenohumeral joint proper. Curves 4 and 6, however, indicate that some of the movement is contributed by the other joints involved.

As abduction proceeds, an increasing amount of movement is contributed by the other joints of the shoulder girdle. In the arc from 30° to 60°, for example, curves 1, 2, 3, and 6 indicate that only about half the movement takes place at the glenohumeral joint. From about 90° of abduction on, curve 1 shows an increasing predominance of motion in the other joints due to increasing inhibition by the capsule and the dwindling lever arm of the deltoid. This contrasts with curves 4 and 5, which indicate a uniform distribution of angular motion.

Shoulder Replacement
Eds.: Kölbel/Helbig/Blauth

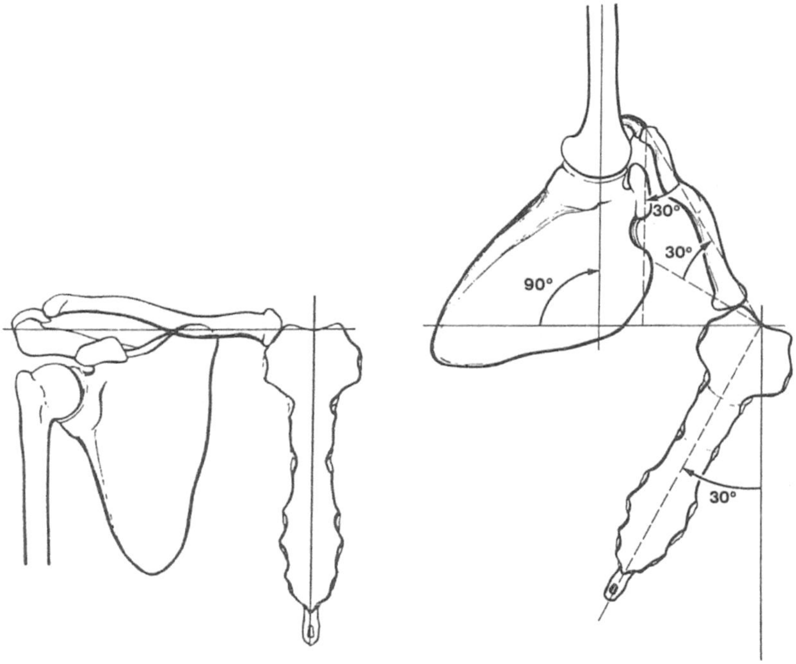


**Fig. 1.** Position of the bones of the shoulder girdle on the frontal plane during extreme abduction of the arm. Only part of the motion takes place at the glenohumeral joint

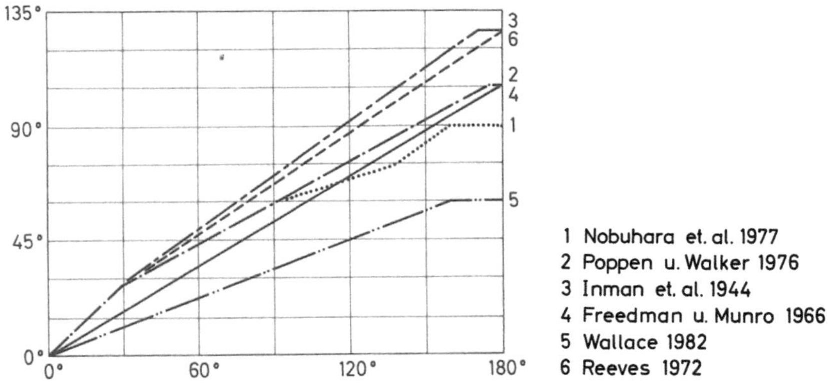


**Fig. 2.** Angular motion at the glenohumeral joint *(vertical axis)* with increasing abduction of the arm *(horizontal axis)*. Results of various authors

As in abduction, the range of motion of the glenohumeral joint about its other axes is limited to approximately 90°, although somewhat larger passive ranges may be possible when the arm is moved by an outside force. This is what makes the design of a prosthetic shoulder joint so difficult. The range of angular motion that can be engineered into a joint prosthesis relates directly to the stability of the joint (its resistance to dislocation) and to the loads that will act on the joint and surrounding bone (Fig. 3).

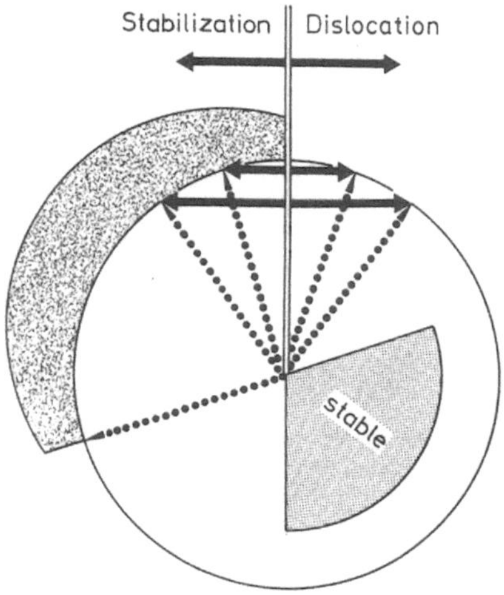


**Fig. 3.** Possible directions of action of joint forces in an unconstrained glenohumeral joint. The joint force directed through the center of the humeral head *(broken line)* must pass through the articular surface of the glenoid; otherwise the joint will dislocate

If an unconstrained design is selected (see also Fig. 8), i.e., a design that reproduces the normal anatomy of the shoulder joint, closure of the joint can be maintained only if all the imposed forces act across the articular surface of the scapular component. Otherwise the joint will dislocate. This means that the directional range of force transmission must be limited to 50°-80° relative to the scapula and to about 150° relative to the humerus. Unfortunately, material technology has not progressed to the point where we are able to design an elastic rim that can replace the function of the glenoid labrum in maintaining reduction. Thus, an unconstrained type of prosthesis is an acceptable option only when muscular function about the shoulder is essentially intact.

If a constrained prosthesis (one with interlocking components) is used in an effort to prevent dislocation (see Figs. 4 and 8), serious technical problems arise: It is not possible to design a simple, durable, constrained ball and socket implant that permits a range of angular motion significantly greater than 90°. Otherwise the neck will impinge on the glenoid rim and place potentially damaging loads on the prosthesis and its bony attachment. If the joint is not ideally positioned, this can occur even at angles less than 90°. More complex designs, such as double ball and socket configurations, have been tried clinically but have not proved successful.

The natural shoulder joint and the unconstrained prosthesis derive their stability from the constant balance that is maintained between the muscular forces acting on the joint. Abduction at the glenohumeral joint is effected mainly by the joint-spanning deltoid muscle (Fig. 5). But the deltoid exerts its greatest pull in an upward direction and would cause superior dislocation of the humeral head from the shallow glenoid were it not opposed by the downward pull of the short rotators.

Different authors report very similar values for the magnitude of the forces acting across the glenohumeral joint (Fig. 6). As the angle of abduction increases, the weight of the arm alone increases the joint force to about 0.8 times the body weight. The joint force decreases again as the arm nears the vertical. When an external weight of only 50 N is held in the laterally extended hand, the estimated force across the joint is approximately 2.5 times the body weight. This load is of the same order of magnitude as at the hip, but it acts across a substantially smaller area of articular

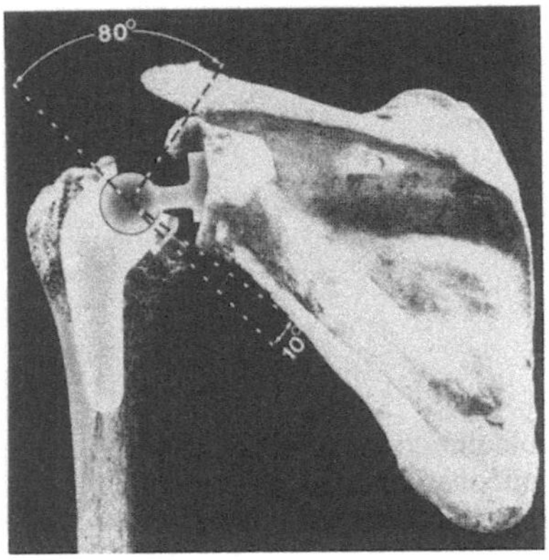


**Fig. 4.** Necessary range of motion for a constrained shoulder prosthesis

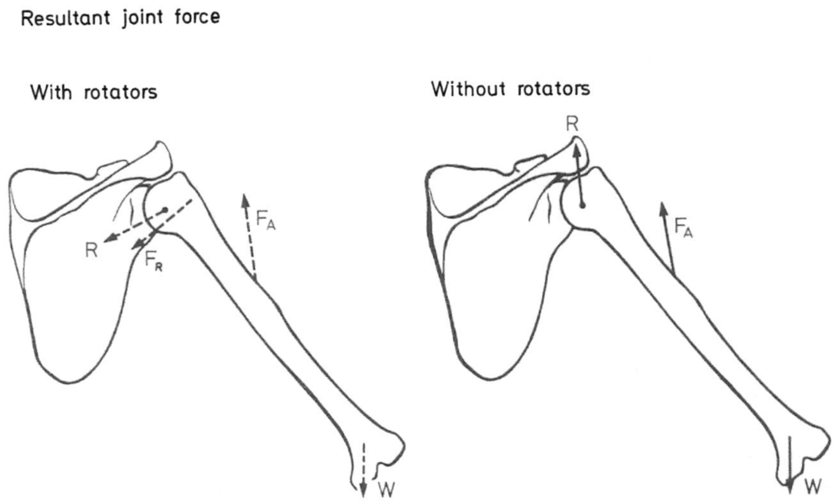


**Fig. 5.** Forces at the natural and unconstrained prosthetic glenohumeral joint. If the abducting deltoid muscle ($F_A$) acts alone *(right)*, the joint will dislocate because the resultant joint force (R) is directed outside the articular surface of the glenoid. If the action of the rotators is added ($F_R$), the resultant force is redirected through the glenoid *(left)*, and closure of the joint is maintained. W Arm weight

contact. Thus we can appreciate the magnitude of the mechanical stresses to which the glenohumeral joint is subjected.

The directions of the joint forces determined by Poppen and Walker are shown in Fig. 7. During elevation of the unloaded arm, the initial joint force is directed downward, the exact direction varying somewhat according to whether the arm is internally or externally rotated. The direction of the force shifts toward the superior edge of the glenoid from about 30° to 60° of abduction, thereafter moving back toward the center of the joint. If this fine muscular control of the force vector is lost, a constrained type of prosthesis is required. A constrained implant would be indicated for partial insufficiency of the rotators and in cases where the joint is not bridged stably enough by the capsule and ligaments.

The resistance to dislocation can be made extremely high in a constrained pros-

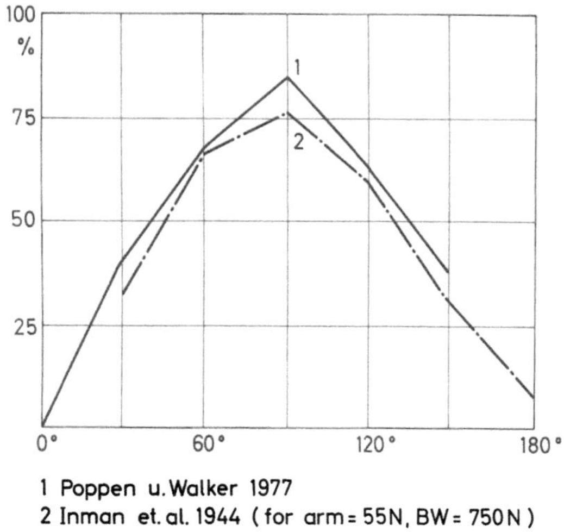


**Fig. 6.** Force at the glenonumeral joint *(vertical axis)* versus angle of abduction *(horizontal axis).* The only load considered is the weight on the arm (55 N, BW=750 N)

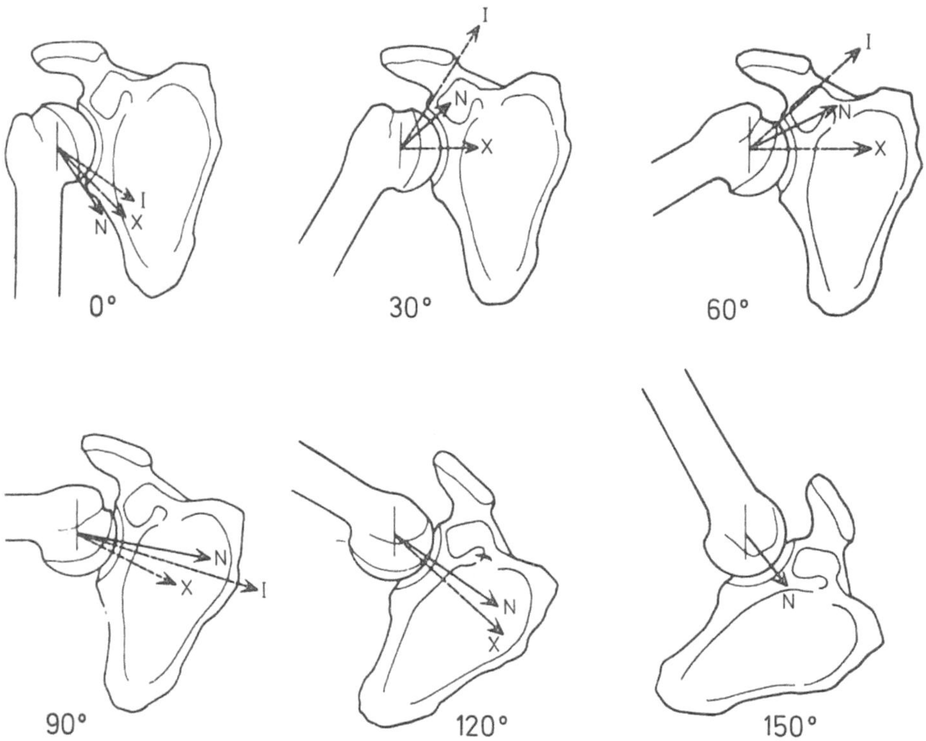


**Fig. 7.** Direction of the forces at the glenohumeral joint with increasing abduction of the arm. The force vectors on the frontal plane for neutral (N), internal (I), and external rotation (X) are shown. (From [6])

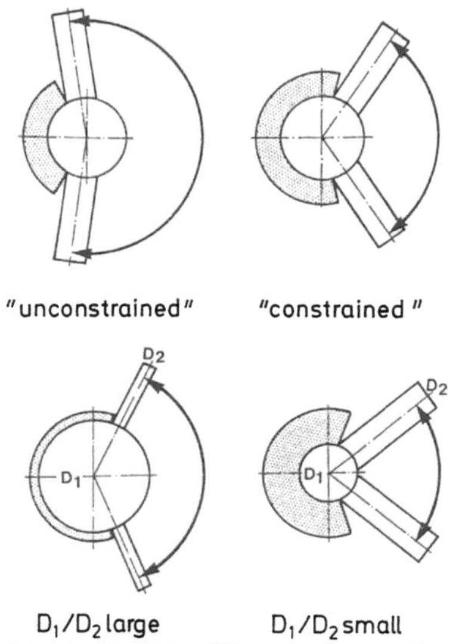


**Fig. 8.** *Top:* Possible angular motions of unconstrained *(left)* and constrained *(right)* prostheses. *Bottom:* Dependence of the angular motion of a constrained prosthesis on the ratio of the head diameter D1 to the neck diameter D2. A large D1/D2 ratio increases the range of motion but compromises the durability and longevity of the joint

thesis. It will be shown, however, that this is not a desirable goal because of the potential stresses that such a device can transmit to the bone. The enclosure angle of the socket (Fig. 8) and the ratio of the neck diameter to the head diameter influence both the range of motion of the joint and its resistance to dislocation. While heavy enclosure of the ball (high degree of constraint) creates maximum opposition to dislocation, it also limits the range of movement. This cannot be offset by decreasing the neck diameter, because the neck must have sufficient mechanical strength. If the neck engages against the socket in the extreme positions, the contact force will be transmitted through a small area; this will lead to plastic deformation at that site and eventually will lessen the resistance of the device to dislocation.

In the Kölbel-Friedebold prosthesis shown in Fig. 9, the geometry and material are designed to permit dislocation at a torque of about 9 Nm - less than that needed to disrupt the bony anchorage of the implant.

Every implant for glenohumeral joint replacement must have a sufficiently large range of motion, must be able to withstand the forces and torques that can develop, and should preserve the approximate anatomic joint center. Its long-term success also depends in large measure on the permanent attachment of the device to the bone. Again, the initial status of the glenohumeral joint may be unfavorable from this standpoint. While the humerus offers ample space for the stable insertion of a prosthesis, the bony volume of the glenoid is very small. Fig. 10 shows the results of photoelastic studies performed in scapular models. One of the models contains no pins, and the other contains two pins representing the anchoring elements of a glenoid prosthesis. The number of lines in the area of the glenoid cavity gives an approximate measure of the magnitude of the stresses that develop in the scapula. It can be seen that stresses are increased substantially by the presence of anchoring pins.

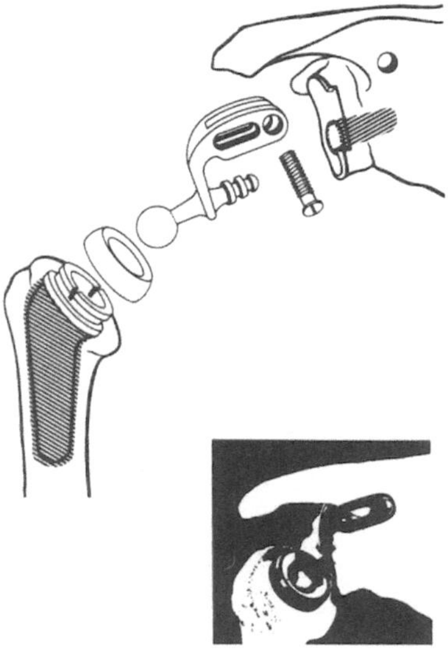

**Fig. 9.** The Kölbel-Friedebold prosthesis. Attachment of the glenoid component is accomplished by an anchoring post and by side struts which fasten to the base of the scapular spine

a

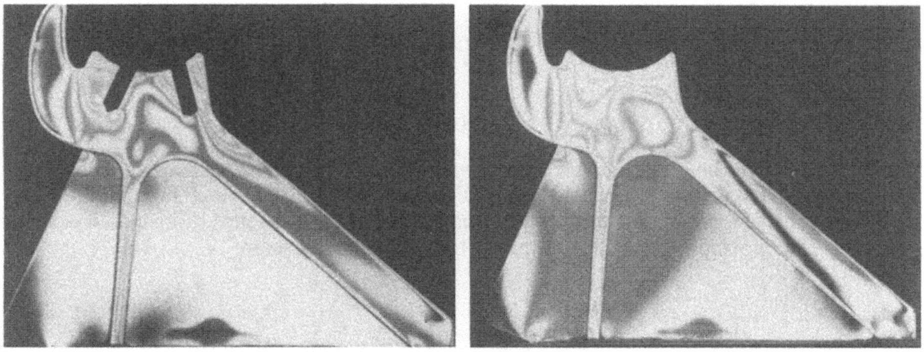

b

**Fig. 10 a,b.** Photoelastic studies of the scapular attachment of a shoulder prosthesis (isochromates in flat models). The number of *dark lines* is a qualitative measure of stress magnitude. We see that substantially higher stresses develop in the presence of an anchored prosthesis **(b)** than in the natural case **(a)**

The schematic drawings in Fig. 11 give a qualitative picture of the mechanical conditions prevalent at the site of attachment of a constrained and unconstrained prosthesis. In the unconstrained joint, in which the possible direction of loading through the glenoid rim is predetermined and in which torques cannot be transmitted, relatively small stresses develop in the bone adjacent to the implant. When dislocation is prevented by a constrained design, impingement of the neck against the glenoid rim causes large torques to act distant from the center of the ball, and the stresses on the bone increase dramatically. Torques of this kind are almost always more disruptive than the stresses produced by pure forces. The bony stresses associated with a constrained prosthesis can be significantly reduced only by providing an additional site of attachment as far as possible from the joint center to serve as a buttress.

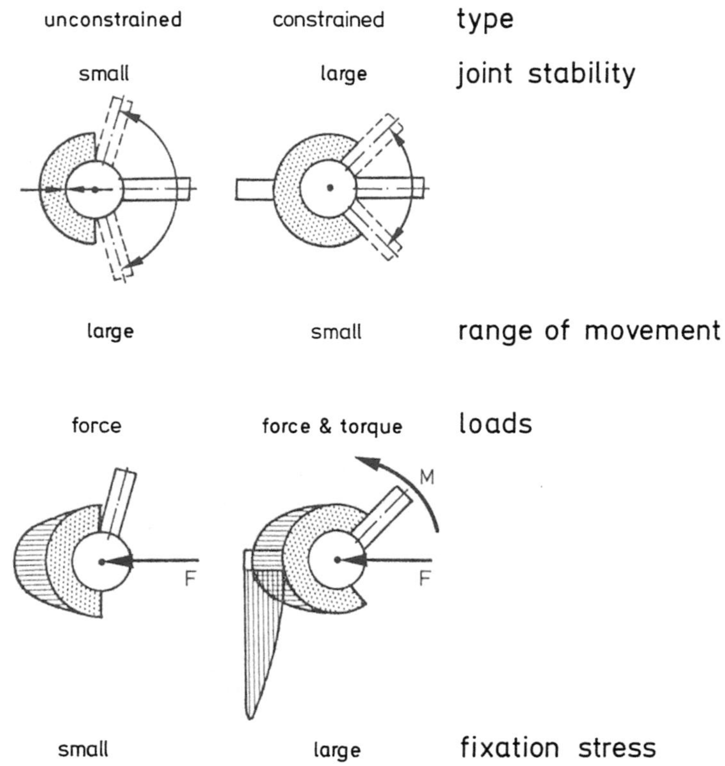


**Fig. 11.** Differences between unconstrained *(left)* and constrained *(right)* shoulder prostheses. The unconstrained design is less resistant to dislocation, has a large range of angular movement, and transmits minimal forces to the bone because of the absence of torque in extreme positions. The opposite statements are true of the constrained design

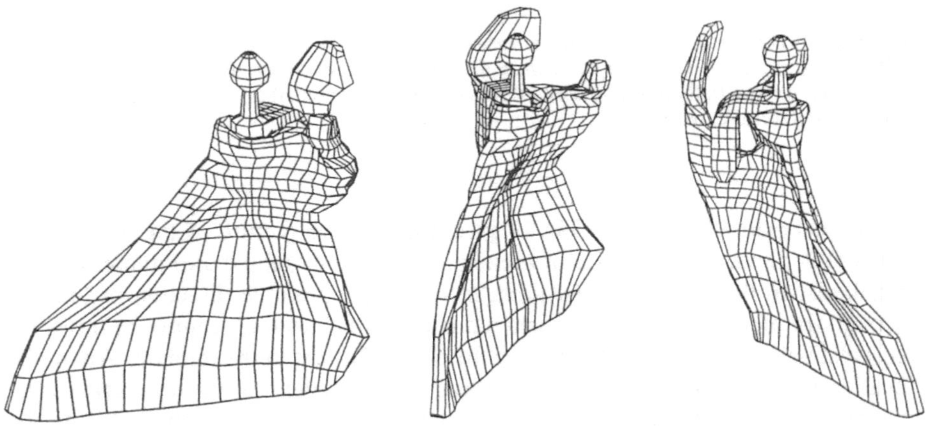

**Fig. 12.** Computer models used to calculate the mechanical stresses on the prosthesis, cement, and surrounding bone (finite element method). These models simulate the Kölbel-Friedebold prosthesis

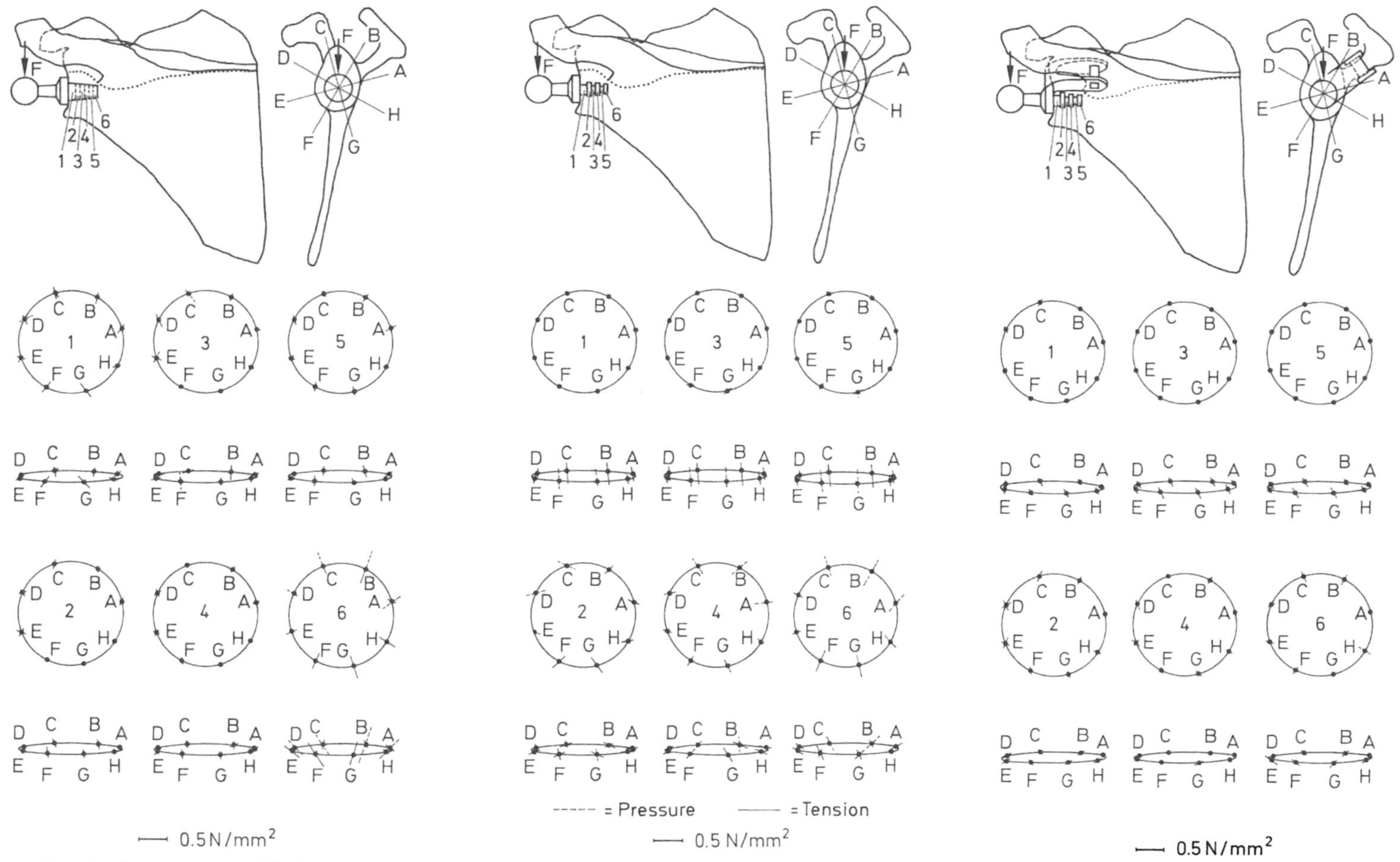


**Fig. 13.** Some results of finite element calculations for shoulder prostheses. Three different prosthetic designs were used: one with a smooth anchoring post *(left)*, one with a stepped post *(center)*, and the Kölbel-Friedebold component with a supplementary buttress. The normal stresses in the cement are shown at different sites along the post (1–6) in cross-section *(circles)* and in a semilateral view *(ellipses)*

The Kölbel-Friedebold prosthesis in Fig. 9 possesses such an attachment at the base of the scapular spine. When this type of device is used, care must be taken that the projecting struts do not interfere with muscular excursions or blood supply, and that they do not cause nerve injury.

Fig. 12 shows a computer-generated model of the scapula with the Kölbel-Friedebold prosthesis in place. This enables us to simulate various conditions of loading and prosthetic attachment.

As an example, Fig. 13 shows the joint loading associated with a weight pulling downward on the arm. The glenoid component in the left part of the figure is anchored by a smooth conical post, that in the center has a stepped post, and that on the right is additionally buttressed by an outrigger fastened to the scapular spine. The stresses on the bone cement around the post are shown in cross-sectional and lateral views at various sites along the post. The increasing post depth 1-6 corresponds to the numbers 1-6 in the lower drawings. The lines illustrate the direction and magnitude of the stresses. Several conclusions may be drawn:

- The magnitude of stresses along the anchoring post is fairly constant (cross-sections 1-5 in left part of figure).
- Higher stresses occur at the tip of the post (cross-section 6 in left part of figure). This pattern is typical of rigid intramedullary fixation and has also been seen in hip and elbow prostheses.
- When the post is stepped for a more stable anchorage (center of figure), local stress concentrations can arise in the cement and bone.
- An extra abutment far from the center of rotation (right part of figure) decreases the stresses by roughly one-third. This finding has been confirmed experimentally.

Table 1 shows experimentally determined values for the dislocation strength and strength of glenoid attachment of various shoulder prostheses. It is important to note that the dislocation and dislodgement of a prosthesis depend not on the forces acting on the prosthesis, but on the moments, or torques, that those forces produce. We see that the attachment of the Kölbel-Friedebold prosthesis can withstand a torque of about 14 Nm in vitro before failure. Post et al. [7] report that the post of a Reese glenoid cup can withstand approximately 30 Nm, without specifying the experimental conditions. We may conclude from this that the dislocation strength of the joint should be limited to a small torque value of no more than 10 Nm by suitable design measures. Otherwise the implant will tend to break from the bone before it dislocates.

**Table 1.** Strength of Attachment and Dislocation Strength (under Torque Loading) of Various Cemented Types of Shoulder Prosthesis

| Author | Attachment strength | Dislocation strength |
|---|---|---|
| Post et al. 1979<br>(Michael Reese model) | 30 Nm<br>2.4-5.8 kN longitud. | 16 Nm |
| Kolbel et al. 1980<br>(Kölbel-Friedebold model) | 14 Nm<br>2 kN longitud.<br>0.5-1 kN transverse | 9 Nm<br>0.7 kN longitud. |
| Beddow and Elloy 1977<br>(Liverpool model) | | 0.9 Nm abduction<br>3.3 Nm rotation |

## Summary

The mechanical status of the scapula may be unfavorable for prosthetic joint replacement. If an unconstrained replacement is proposed to restore only the function of the joint itself, satisfactory solutions are possible, as indicated by clinical results with several types of prosthesis. But if it is necessary to restore or replace the function of soft-tissue structures like the capsule, muscles, or ligaments in addition to the joint itself, we can, for the forseeable future, expect only compromise solutions whose mechanical and clinical results are less than satisfactory.

## References

1. Beddow FH, Elloy MA (1977) The Liverpool total replacement for the glenohumeral joint. In: Joint replacement of the upper limb. The Justitution of Mechanical Engineers, Conference Publication No 5, pp 21-25
2. Freedman L, Munro RR (1966) Abduction of the arm in the scapular plane: Scapular and glenohumeral movements. J Bone Joint Surg [Am] 48: 1503-1510
3. Inman VT, Saunders JB, Abbott LC (1944) Observations on the function of the shoulder joint. J Bone Joint Surg 26: 1-40
4. Kölbel R, Rohlmann A, Bergmann G (1980) Experimentelle Untersuchungen zur Verankerung einer Schultergelenkendoprothese. In: Jäger M, Hackenbroch MH, Refior HJ (Hrsg) Endprothese, Endoprothetik und Biomechanik der Gelenke. Thieme, Stuttgart, S 54-61
5. Poppen NK, Walker PS (1976) Normal and abnormal motion of the shoulder. J Bone Joint Surg [Am] 58: 195-201
6. Poppen NK, Walker PS (1978) Forces at the glenohumeral joint in abduction. Clin Orthop 135: 165-170
7. Post M, Jablon M, Miller H, Singh M (1979) Constrained shoulder joint replacement: A critical review. Clin Orthop 144: 135-149
8. Reeves B, Jobbins B, Flowers M (1972) Biomechanical problems in the developement of a total shoulder endoprosthesis. (Proc Br Orthop Res Soc) J Bone Joint Surg [Br] 54: 193
9. Rohlmann A, Mössner U, Bergmann G (1985) Rechnerische Spannungsanalyse am endoprothetisch versorgten Schulterblatt. In: Refior HJ, Plitz W, Jäger M, Hackenbroch MH (Hrsg) Biomechanik der gesunden und kranken Schulter. Thieme, Stuttgart, S 198-202

# Alternative Procedures and Indications

# Results of Resection Arthroplasty and the Benjamin Double Osteotomy

K. Tillmann and D. Braatz

When conservative treatment options have been exhausted in the rheumatoid shoulder, our policy at the Orthopedic Department of the Rheumatology Hospital in Bad Bramstedt has been to use synovectomy, the Benjamin double osteotomy [1], and our own technique of resection arthroplasty [4] with approximately equal frequencies.

## Patient Selection

Lacking other guidelines, our criteria for patient selection are based essentially on our own experience and therefore cannot be considered binding.

*Synovectomies* are used to treat a congruent joint with a salvagable gliding surface that shows obvious clinical signs of active inflammation. Radiographic findings and clinical features are equally important for patient selection. The final decision, however, is sometimes made at the operating table. At present we feel that large cysts and significant secondary degenerative changes contraindicate synovectomy.

With advanced joint destruction, synovectomy alone is no longer adequate, although we consider it a necessary adjunct in most reconstructive procedures, if only for the purpose of arthrolysis. We have found *double osteotomy* and *resection arthroplasty* to be of substantial value in late-stage cases, following the disappointing results of total shoulder replacements.

Our criteria for selecting one procedure over the other relate mainly to the patient's willingness and readiness for operative treatment and to individual functional demands. In patients who are cooperative - especially patients known to be cooperative from earlier therapy - we favor resection arthroplasty. The candidates for this procedure often maintain relatively high functional demands despite significant disability, a characteristic which distinguishes them from cases in which we recommend double osteotomy. For the patient, the difference between the two procedures lies less in the stress of the operation than in the rigors of postoperative care. These are minimal after the double osteotomy but can be formidable after the resection arthroplasty.

At one time we considered age to be an important factor in patient selection, tending to favor the double osteotomy in older patients and the resection arthroplasty in younger ones. The follow-up studies of D. Braatz finally convinced us that this viewpoint was unfounded (see Table 1).

## Operative Technique and Postoperative Care

Briefly, the double osteotomy of Benjamin [1] is performed through an anterior approach. An osteotomy is made through the neck of the scapula, and the proximal humeral metaphysis is osteotomized at the level of the surgical neck, in both cases

Shoulder Replacement
Eds.: Kölbel/Helbig/Blauth

sparing the posterior periosteum. Synovectomy is done only to the extent necessary for satisfactory exposure. Postoperatively the arm is immobilized in a Desault bandage for 2–4 days, and thereafter in a sling. The sling is worn for another 6–10 days, at the patient's discretion. The patient decides how he will resume use of the arm, and this should be done strictly according to tolerance. Exercises are contraindicated.

The resection arthroplasty is done through a transacromial approach and involves detachment of most of the rotator cuff. A radical synovectomy is performed, and the head of the humerus is reshaped and covered with lyophilized dura. Then the rotator cuff is reconstructed as needed and reattached to the humerus under physiologic tension. Tillmann, unlike Gariepy [2], places great importance on avoiding further reduction of the already damaged glenoid so that the center of rotation will not be displaced too far medially. He also recommends reducing the size of the humeral head to facilitate reconstruction of the usually deficient rotator cuff, and increasing retroversion by about 10° over the physiologic value to lessen the risk of dislocation. An abduction splint is worn for about 6 weeks postoperatively, and only passive motion from the splint is allowed initially. This is followed by a program of active physiotherapy lasting several months or in some cases up to one year.

## Results

The results of both procedures were studied and compiled by Braatz within the framework of a doctoral thesis for the Hamburg University School of Medicine.

It is tempting the compare the results of the procedures with each other (Table 1), but this would not be valid because of our differential approach to patient selection. A comparison would be unfairly biased against the double osteotomy, because we tended to use this procedure in our less cooperative candidates (see above).

In terms of pain relief (Table 2), the results of the resection arthroplasty were better than we had expected after we had almost abandoned prosthetic replacement in favor of this procedure.

We did, of course, expect that the resection arthroplasty would improve the range of shoulder motion (Table 3). Indeed, this was the main objective of the procedure, whereas the double osteotomy was intended only to relieve pain and perhaps ameliorate the local inflammatory response – an effect that was consistently obtained.

The positive effect on active range of motion is also apparent in the improvement of everyday function (Table 4), which determines the patient's level of self-sufficiency. In this respect the results of the resection arthroplasty were superior even to those we had obtained earlier with replacement arthroplasty.

The complications are listed in Table 5. In percentage terms, the numbers are not inconsequential. We believe, however, that the complication rate can be decreased as more experience is gained.

The subjective ratings by the patients (Table 6) clearly reflect their different initial conditions and attitudes, which were important criteria in our differential patient selection (see above).

**Table 1.** Resection-Interposition Arthroplasties (RIAP) and Double Osteotomies (DO) of the Shoulder Joint Performed at Bad Bramstedt from 1981-1984

| | RIAP | DO |
|---|---|---|
| Diagnosis | Rheumatoid arthritis | Rheumatoid arthritis |
| Patients (n) | 22<br>20 women, 2 men | 24<br>15 women, 9 men |
| Joints | R 11, L 11 | R 11, L 13 |
| Age (years) | 54 (31-74) | 54 (39-72) |
| Follow-up (months) | 30 (6-57) | 29 (14-44) |

**Table 2.** Pain Before and After Operation. 0 = None, 1 = Mild, 2 = Moderate, 3 = Severe

| | RIAP | | DO | |
|---|---|---|---|---|
| n | 22 | | 24 | |
| | Before | After | Before | After |
| Pain | 2.51 | 0.82 | 2.34 | 1.51 |

**Table 3.** Ranges of Active Motion Before and After Operation

| | RIAP | | DO | |
|---|---|---|---|---|
| n | 22 | | 24 | |
| Active motion | Before | After | Before | After |
| Flexion | 65° | 97° | 97° | 95° |
| Abduction | 56° | 90° | 69° | 77° |
| Humeroglenoid abduction | | 70° | | 49° |

**Table 4.** Ability to Perform Everyday Functions Before and After Operation. 0 = Easy, 1 = Difficult, 2 = Incomplete, 3 = Impossible

| | RIAP | | DO | |
|---|---|---|---|---|
| n | 22 | | 24 | |
| Function | Before | After | Before | After |
| Reaching behind head and neck | 2.50 | 1.32 | 2.38 | 1.67 |
| Reaching behind back ("apron tying") | 1.96 | 0.91 | 2.17 | 1.33 |

**Table 5.** Complications of Resection Arthroplasty (RIAP) and Double Osteotomy (DO) and Their Treatment (in Parentheses)

| | RIAP | DO |
|---|---|---|
| n | 22 | 24 |
| | Instability<br>2<br>(1 arthrodesis) | Nonunion<br>1<br>(1 RIAP) |

**Table 6.** Subjective Rating of Both Procedures by the Patients. 0 = Not Satisfied, 1 = Undecided, 2 = Satisfied, 3 = Very Satisfied

| | RIAP | DO |
|---|---|---|
| n | 22 | 24 |
| Rating by patient | 2.41 | 1.67 |

## Summary

It is our impression that both procedures basically fulfilled their purpose and the expectations placed in them.

We were pleasantly surprised by the improved range of motion seen in some patients after double osteotomy, but we were somewhat disappointed by the level of pain relief. The reasons were discussed.

The overall results of the resection arthroplasty were better than we had anticipated before the study. We feel that this procedure offers an effective alternative to shoulder replacement arthroplasty, as it does, for example, in the elbow joint [3]. The procedure is inappropriate when bone stock has been so greatly reduced by destruction and cyst formation that reshaping of the femoral head is no longer feasible. Also, a reasonably functional and reparable rotator cuff must be present that the surgeon is able to identify and mobilize.

Giant cysts in the humeral head are a relatively common obstacle to reconstruction that have spoiled the result of many a late synovectomy. Even the grafting of autologous bone chips cannot solve all problems in this regard, and there have been cases where we were compelled to perform a total shoulder replacement as our only recourse.

## References

1. Benjamin A (1974) Double osteotomy of the shoulder. Scand J Rheumatol 3: 65
2. Gariepy R (1977) Gleniodectomy in the repair of the rheumatoid shoulder. J Bone Joint Surg [Br] 59: 122
3. Thabe H, Tillmann K (1983) Spätergebnisse von Resektionsarthroplastiken der oberen Extremität im Vergleich zur Alloarthroplastik. Orthop Prax 9: 662-670
4. Tillmann K (1982) Die operative Behandlung des rheumatischen Schultergelenkes. Chir Prax 30: 485-489

# Indications, Technique, and Results of Shoulder Arthrodesis

P. Raunio

Although the shoulder joint is affected in more than 50% of patients hospitalized for chronic rheumatoid arthritis at the Rheumatism Foundation Hospital in Heinola, Finland, this joint has traditionally been somewhat neglected. Surgery has not offered any clear solutions. In the past 10 years, with refinements in replacement arthroplasty, the topic has again become a focus of attention. Arthrodesis has become less popular, and today some enthusiasts of shoulder replacement are asking whether an indication for arthrodesis still exists at all. We know, however, that all shoulder prostheses cannot function indefinitely, and that this limits their application in younger patients. Also, we must remember that arthrodesis can be very difficult if not impossible following the removal of a prosthesis.

It is a fact that joint replacement arthroplasty has almost entirely supplanted arthrodesis in recent years. Some colleagues consider shoulder arthrodesis to be nothing more than a salvage procedure for failed arthroplasties. Given the poor results of improperly positioned arthrodeses, this view is understandable. The position of the arthrodesis is of crucial importance.

To assess the value of arthrodesis, we conducted a follow-up study of 39 patients with 41 shoulder fusions performed from 1957 to 1977 [1, 3]. By September, 1984, we had performed a total of 63 shoulder arthrodeses, or 22 operations after the conclusion of our study. At our center, too, replacement arthroplasty has tended to supplant arthrodesis in the last 5 years, and the indications for arthrodesis have been correspondingly limited.

The average age of our follow-up population was 36 years. The duration of symptoms, at 12 years, was relatively long. The length of follow-up was 6 years, which is presumed to be adequate for assessing long-term results.

We shall not go into the details of the operative technique, other than to note that we ordinarily use three compression screws: one placed through the acromion into the humeral head, one through the humeral head into the glenoid, and a third through the coracoid process into the humeral head. No cases of infection were seen, but we saw four instances of nonunion at the glenohumeral joint. These did not require reoperation, because the complaints were mild. Two other patients experienced mild pain in the acromioclavicular joint. On the whole, it was surprising that this joint caused complaints so rarely, even when obvious radiographic changes were visible. Overall pain relief was good, as we had expected.

It is also interesting to note how the arthrodesis affected the overall range of shoulder motion. We found that the operation significantly improved overall mobility in flexion and abduction. Records on rotational mobility were unfortunately so vauge that they could not be evaluated. We know, however, that rotation is the movement most greatly limited by arthrodesis.

On average, the range of shoulder abduction and flexion increased from 100° to 160°. The apparent paradox of arthrodesis improving mobility is due to the freedom of motion that exists in the thoracoscapular joint, which is appreciably better in younger patients than in the elderly.

Shoulder Replacement
Eds.: Kölbel/Helbig/Blauth

But one should not dwell too strongly on quantitative data, which do not necessarily reflect the actual result. The main criterion of success is functional outcome. An operation is accepted by the patient only if it improves his ability to perform everyday tasks. Success in achieving this goal depends chiefly on an optimum position of the arthrodesis.

The average position of the arthrodesis was 55° abduction, 25° flexion, and an internal rotation allowing hand-to-mouth movement, i.e., about 25°-30°. The degree of internal rotation should be such that the arm is able to hang freely at the side. If the upper arm is positioned in, say, 30° abduction and 30° flexion, this means that the forearm must be brought onto the horizontal plane to obtain 30° of internal rotation. Three important motor functions were measured: 1) hand to mouth, 2) hand to buttocks, and 3) hand behind the neck. Fifteen patients could perform all 3 movements; 13 could perform only 1. All patients were able to eat, dress, and manage their personal hygiene. All believed that they had benefitted from the operation.

Bony consolidation is successfully accomplished in most cases. We immobilize the arm on a light plastic splint weighing only 750 g, which is worn for about 8-12 weeks. The splint is custom fabricated and is easily placed in the desired position.

Today our position of choice for arthrodesis of the shoulder is 30° abduction, 30° flexion, and 30° internal rotation (Fig. 1). This formula is easily remembered, and the position is consistent with the recommendations of Rowe [2] and our own experience. Greater abduction is unnecessary and can be disadvantageous. The same is true of hyperflexion. Both create a protrusion of the scapula and often result in painful shoulder muscles.

If we know that prosthetic replacement usually gives a better functional result, it is reasonable to ask why we still need arthrodeses. At our center, however, shoulder prostheses have not made arthrodesis obsolete by any means, and it is unlikely that they will do so in the future.

Our indications for arthrodesis are as follows:

1. Severe destruction of the shoulder joint in patients under 50 years of age.

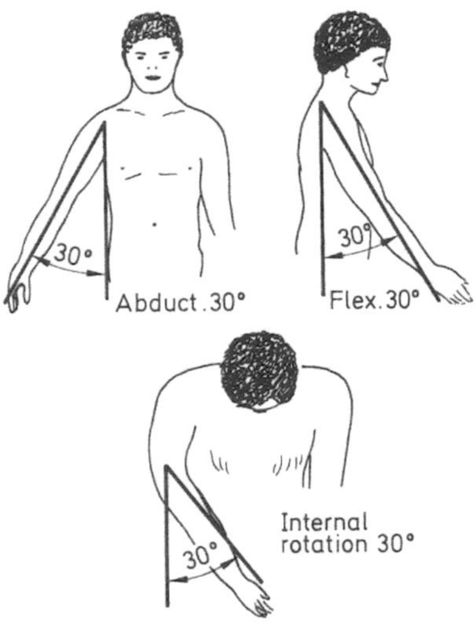


**Fig. 1.** Recommended position for arthrodesis of the shoulder

If the contralateral joint will require operation later, we try to insert a prosthesis at the earliest possible opportunity.

2. If both shoulder joints require operation, we perform a replacement arthroplasty on the right (stronger) side and an arthrodesis on the left side. This ensures that the patient will have a serviceable hand for life.
3. In manual laborers in whom a prosthesis would quickly loosen, we prefer to perform an arthrodesis.

## References

1. Raunio P (1981) Arthrodesis of the shoulder joint in rheumatoid arthritis. Reconstr Surg Traumatol 18: 48-54
2. Rowe CW (1974) Re-evaluation of the position of the arm in arthrodesis of the shoulder in adult. J Bone Joint Surg [Am] 56: 913-922
3. Rybka V, Raunio P, Vainio K (1979) Arthrodesis of the shoulder in rheumatoid arthritis. A review of forty-one cases. J Bone Joint Surg [Br] 61: 155-158

# Selection of Patients for Shoulder Replacement

R. Kölbel

Shoulder replacement arthroplasty is always an elective procedure. The need for shoulder surgery depends on the diagnosis. If surgery is considered necessary, the decision to proceed with replacement arthroplasty must be freely made by the physician and patient. Accordingly, high demands are placed on the safety of the procedure and its result.

Why replace the shoulder joint?

Three diagnostic groups can be identified:

Group A: stiff, painful shoulder from *deformation or destruction of the articular surfaces*

Group B: unstable and painful shoulder with soft and/or hard *tissue defects*

Group C: fractures with destruction or potential avascular necrosis of the humeral head *(trauma).*

The therapeutic objectives in these groups are:

- pain relief
- stability
- active mobility.

These goals are attainable only to a limited degree with conventional methods. The contributions of Tillmann and Raunio demonstrate how good the results of alternative procedures can be.

Experience in the area of alloarthroplasty is now available and will be addressed in this volume.

Now is the time to make available experience a basis for broader application, and this brings us to the question of *patient selection.*

The diagnoses contained in the three categories defined above are not very numerous and are seen time and again in reviews of large series. I will use some of these diagnoses to illustrate the process that is involved in patient selection, limiting my considerations to cases that fall in category of group A (deformation or destruction of the joint surfaces) or group B (shoulders with tissue defects).

In the process of patient selection, the following questions have to be addressed in the order indicated:

What is bothering the patient?
What does the patient want?
What is causing the condition?
What is the prognosis without surgical treatment?
What surgical options are available?
What can they achieve?

If replacement arthroplasty is being considered, the following additional questions have to be addressed:

Are the muscular stabilizers and motors intact, functioning, or reparable?
Is the bone length preserved?
Is the attachment of a prosthesis feasible?
What are the options for salvage or conversion?

Shoulder Replacement
Eds.: Kölbel/Helbig/Blauth

Is the patient motivated and cooperative?

Do any of the following contraindications exist:

- radiation damage or immune deficiency (LE)
- neuroarthropathy (e.g., syringomyelia)
- infection (osteomyelitis, Tuberculosis)
- compensation claims (in some cases)
- psychiatric disorders.

Now as in the past, dissatisfaction with existing treatments has stimulated an ongoing search for new approaches. Such efforts have existed for many years (see Chap. 1), especially in cases where surgical treatment is mandatory, such as malignant tumors and fractures which have a poor functional prognosis. Accordingly, we have been able to acquire the greatest amount of experience in these types of indications. For situations in which surgery is not mandatory, we must draw on experience that is well founded and is gained 1) with due consideration of *theoretical principles* (biomechanics of the shoulder, general principles of replacement arthroplasty), 2) with use of and regard for the correct *method* (operative technique, rehabilitation), and 3) with use of an appropriate *implant* (design, material, method of attachment).

In all three points, the shoulder joint presents unique problems which distinguish it from other joints such as the hip. The differences are less qualitative (wear, interfacial problems, material considerations) than quantitative and relate to the fact that the shoulder joint derives most of its stability from soft tissues, and that it offers little in the way of preformed bony cavities for the attachment of prosthetic devices.

Only when one understands the biomechanics of the shoulder, tailors the operative approach and postoperative care accordingly, and has an implant whose capabilities are known and which will not itself create problems, can one begin to define more clearly the types of shoulder conditions that will benefit from prosthetic joint replacement.

Let us now trace the process of patient selection, taking a case from group A as an example (Fig. 1 a,b):

A 58-year-old woman with posttraumatic necrosis of the humeral head is bothered most by pain and limited motion. She wants pain relief and better mobility.

The radiograph shows that the condition is caused by deformation of the humeral joint surface, leading to incongruity. The accompanying inflammatory changes lead to pain and finally to contracture.

The prognosis without surgery is that the pain may subside in a few years, with no improvement in range of motion.

Of the surgical options that exist, double osteotomy is unsuitable because of the incongruent joint surfaces. Arthrodesis would be possible, would alleviate pain, restore stability, and provide an acceptable range of pain-free motion. But the patient refuses this option. Resection arthroplasty is possible and would probably relieve pain, but it would not provide the desired amount of stability and active movement.

Because previous experience indicates that replacement arthroplasty offers superior functional results in this setting, it is considered.

Going down the list of questions, we note that the muscles are intact, and that the bone length is not preserved but is restorable by the arthroplasty. Prosthetic attachment is feasible.

Conversion to a resection arthroplasty or arthrodesis is possible in the event of implant removal, with the results that one would expect from those procedures.

The patient is highly motivated and cooperative. No contraindications exist. In this setting prospects are excellent for achieving pain relief, stability, and active mobility. Less is accomplished with the alternative procedures, and so an indication exists for replacement arthroplasty.

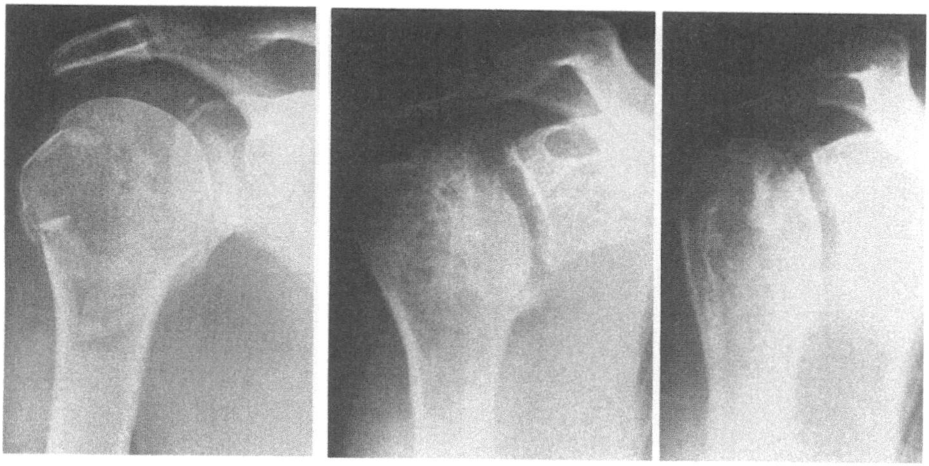

a b

**Fig. 1 a,b.** Woman 58 years of age with posttraumatic avascular necrosis of the humeral head. The shoulder is stiff and painful

It is apparent from the large series of Neer et al. [1] that the gains of active motion and power parallel each other, and that they are better in patients with degenerative changes than in patients with old fractures, roughly in the sequence osteoarthritis of the shoulder, arthritis of dislocation, rheumatoid arthritis, old fracture.

If the prerequisite conditions are not met, especially with regard to the muscles and tendon cuff, the prospects for a functional recovery are limited. Repair of the rotator cuff demands caution during postoperative care, and goals should be modified in line with Neer's principle of "limited-goals" rehabilitation. According to Neer, stability takes precedence over range of motion when significant muscle damage has occurred.

Our next example involves a 65-year-old man with osteoarthritis of both hips and shoulders from the same diagnostic category:

The patient is bothered mainly by stiffness in both shoulders; pain is a lesser complaint. Mobility is his main concern. The condition is caused by a polyarticular osteoarthritis with bilateral loss of articular cartilage, inflammatory changes, and contractures. The condition would not improve without surgery (Fig. 2).

Concerning therapeutic options, resection arthroplasty was not offered, and arthrodesis was inconsistent with the demand for mobility.

The prerequisites for prosthetic replacement - intact, functioning muscles, intact bone length, feasibility of prosthetic attachment, conversion options, motivation - were all present, and no contraindications existed.

The alternative procedures offered less favorable results, and so the decision for replacement arthropathy was made. A constrained prosthesis was used in this patient.

A 59-year-old woman (Fig. 3) with rheumatoid arthritis was bothered most by limited motion and less by pain, although radiographic findings and good passive motion under anesthesia implied that pain was the major cause of the restricted motion. The patient mainly wanted a better range of shoulder movement. Her condition would not have improved without surgery.

Of the alternative procedures, arthrodesis was not considered because both shoulders and both elbows were involved by arthritis. Double osteotomy would not have been possible, nor would resection arthroplasty. It is doubtful whether the prospects for functional recovery would have been as good with these procedures as with prosthetic replacement.

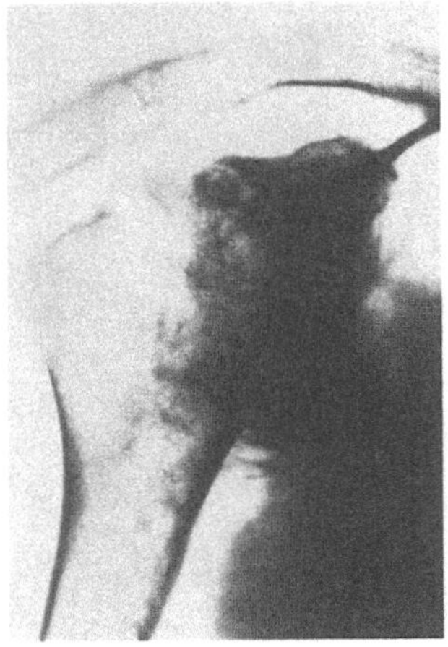

**Fig. 2.** Man 65 years of age with a stiff, painful shoulder due to osteoarthritis

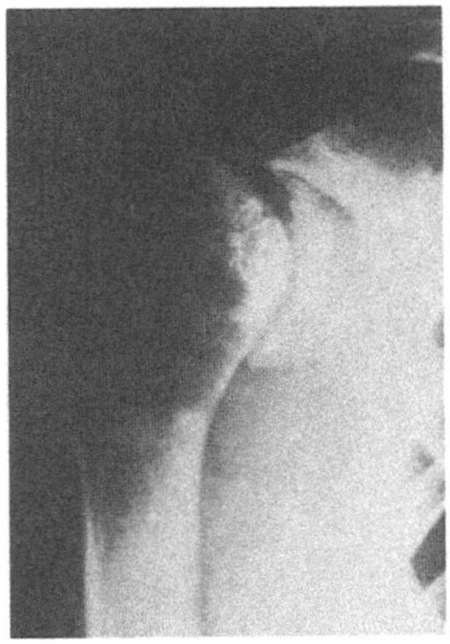

**Fig. 3.** Woman 59 years of age with shoulder pain and stiffness due to rheumatoid arthritis

This case satisfied all the prerequisites for replacement arthroplasty. Today it is clear that joint replacement and subsequent rehabilitation offered excellent prospects for pain relief, stability, and active motion. At the time the patient was operated, in 1976, a constrained type of prosthesis was used.

In the series of Neer et al. [1] and of Post et al. [2], arthritis of dislocation is considered an indication for total shoulder arthroplasty. This indication is not commonly recognized outside the United States.

In group B (shoulders with tissue defects), the patient selection process is somewhat different because of the necessity of surgical treatment. Again, the use of prostheses is elective but is highly desirable because of the opportunity for functional recovery.

A somewhat different list of questions is applied in a 36-year-old man with a chondrosarcoma: What is left after an adequate tumor resection, and what function can the patient expect?

Significant sacrifice of bone length in this patient, with loss of the rotator attachments, left an unstable shoulder with limited active motion and moderate complaints. This condition could not be expected to resolve without treatment (Fig. 4 a-d).

Of the available therapeutic options, arthrodesis would require the insertion of a massive bone graft to avoid excessive shortening and deformity. The result would be a stable shoulder with a limited range of motion. Replacement of the upper end of the humerus with a vascularized fibular graft could preserve arm length, but shoulder stability would be compromised, and its range of active motion would be seriously limited. The experience of Neer and others indicates that hemiarthroplasty should be given consideration in this setting.

As for prerequisites, we find that reconstruction of the rotator cuff and its insertions would be difficult. Bone length can be corrected with an appropriate implant. Prosthetic attachment is feasible. Removal of the implant is possible as an eventual option.

In this situation the prospects for stability and active motion are limited. Postoperative care cannot be directed toward achieving full mobility, and the first priority is stability.

Previous experience demonstrates that hemiarthroplasty can accomplish more than the alternative procedures, and it is indicated in the present case.

The use of implants in shoulders with irreparable muscular defects, and in which constrained prostheses could preserve the shape and stability of the shoulder, is dis-

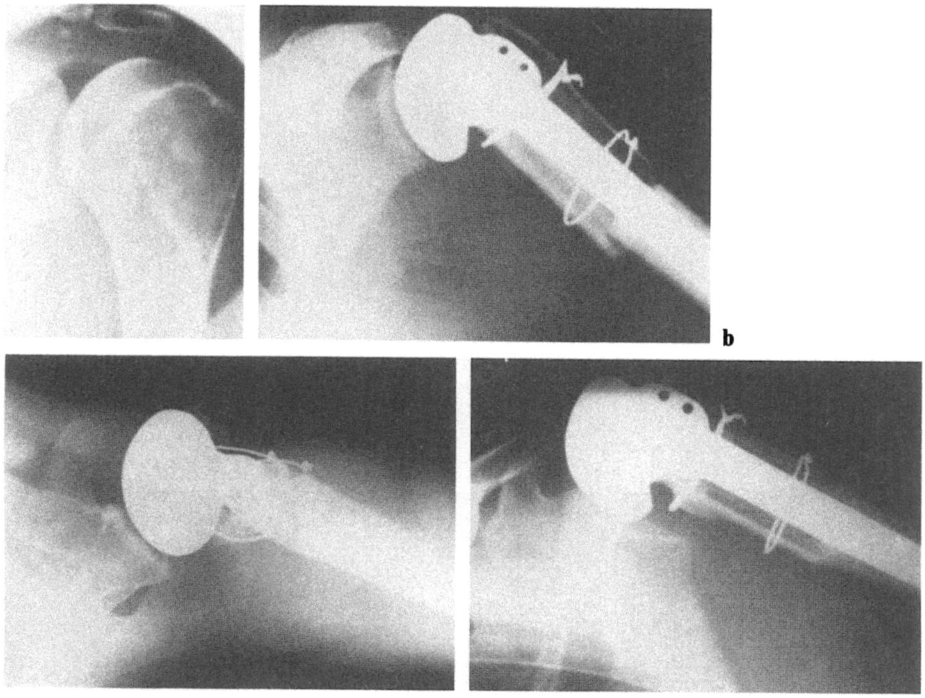

a b c d

**Fig. 4a-d.** Man 36 years of age with chondrosarcoma **(a)** 2 months after **(b)** and 2 years after replacement of the proximal humerus with a Neer prosthesis, cancellous bone, and a free vascularized fibular graft **(c,d)**. Note the upward subluxation of the prosthesis

cussed elsewhere in this volume. Constrained joint replacement is still not a proven treatment.

I would include patients with cuff-tear arthropathy in the group B category. The presence of a massive, old defect of the rotator cuff with muscular atrophy and extensive distortion of the subacromial space would tax the capabilities of any procedure. It will probably be several years before we can say with certainty whether an implant can provide stability in cases of this type. If we are to avoid discrediting the already proven method of unconstrained joint replacement, we should not regard this condition as a valid indication at the present time (Fig. 5 a,b).

The category of shoulders with tissue defects also includes shoulders that have had previous surgery. Due to ignorance of the function of the shoulder joint, a certain hopelessness, or perhaps lack of a better method, surgeons continue to resect tissue from the shoulder without a compelling reason and without proceeding with a proper resection arthroplasty.

Patients in this category, illustrated here by a 74-year-old woman, are bothered by pain and lack of active mobility (Fig. 4, page 192). These are consequences of instability. The patient in this case wants less pain and more stability, and if possible an increased range of active motion. The only alternative procedure worth considering, arthrodesis, was refused.

Is replacement arthroplasty possible in this case, where the rotators and a large portion of the deltoid have been sacrificed in a previous operation?

Soft-tissue reconstruction, if at all possible, would be extremely difficult and incomplete. The bone length is deficient but could be reconstructed. All other prerequisites in this patient are satisfied reasonably well.

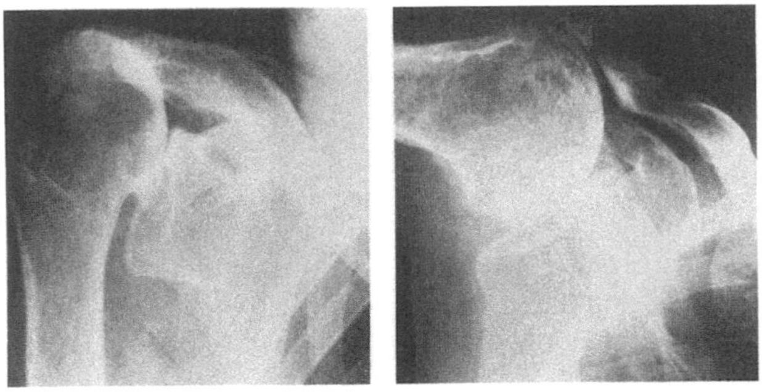

a b

**Fig. 5a,b.** Long-standing case of cuff-tear arthropathy

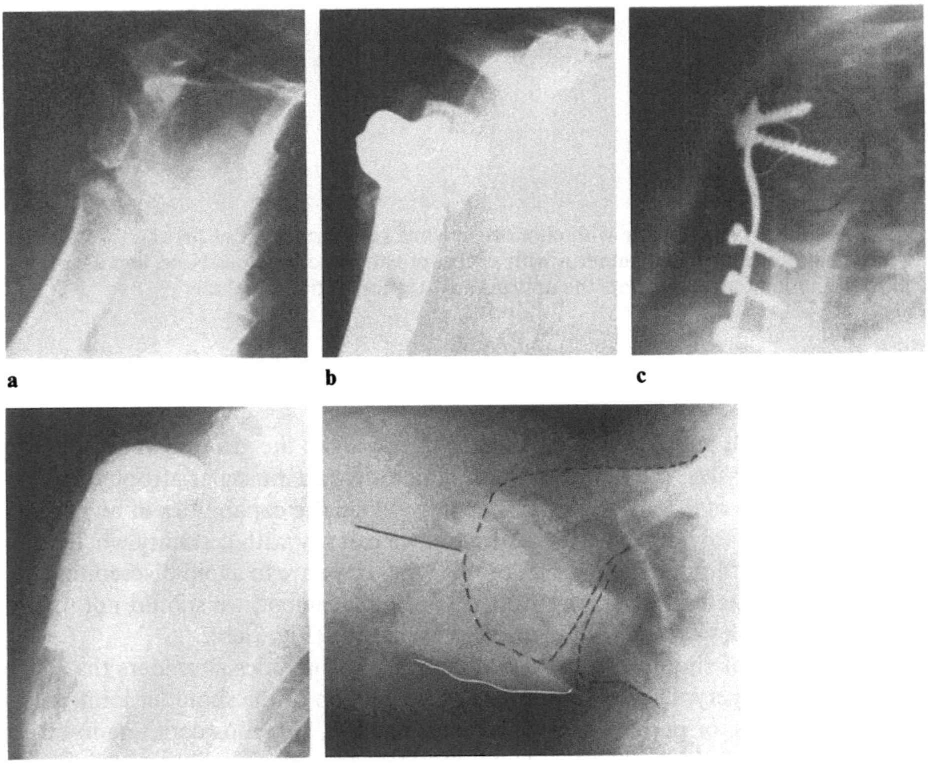

a b c

d e

**Fig. 6a-e.** Woman 58 years of age with a 3-part fracture and sequelae to attempted internal fixation - removal of fragments and "replacement" by bone cement.

Viewing the possibilities critically, one would have to say that arthroplasty with a proven unconstrained prosthesis would at best offer a very limited prospect of success. The same can be said of hemiarthroplasty, which should have been combined initially with the humeral head resection.

I would like to relate the case of another previously operated shoulder with tissue defects, in which we can readily identify the point at which reconstruction with a prosthetic humeral head replacement would have been feasible (Fig. 6 a-e). Aside from other technical possibilites in this fracture, once the decision had been made to resect the humeral head, it would have been possible to preserve the tuberosities and reconstruct the humeral head with a long-stem prosthesis, creating a very good prospect for functional recovery.

A 76-year-old woman who underwent a previous humeral head replacement (Fig. 5, page 193) is now bothered by severe pains. These are due partly to strain on the stabilizing muscles of the shoulder girdle and partly to displacement of the head of the prosthesis when active motion is attempted.

The causes are loss of the rotator origins and deficient restoration of the length of the humerus.

The prognosis is no change without further surgery.

Alternative procedures do not appear feasible, and arthrodesis would be a very involved procedure in this patient.

A major prerequisite for a successful unconstrained replacement, an intact muscular apparatus, is lacking, and its reconstruction would be difficult or impossible. Bone length is not preserved, and there is a danger that the humerus will fracture on removal of the prosthesis. Reconstruction with a long-stem implant would be possible.

The poor soft-tissue status in this case precludes the use of proven unconstrained implants, and so an indication does not exist for this type of reconstruction.

This case finally was managed by revision with a constrained prosthesis.

## Summary

*Unconstrained* joint replacement with proven implants and techniques is used in cases where deformity or destruction of the articular surfaces seriously impairs their congruity, and where the active muscular stabilizers and motors of the shoulder joint are either intact or amenable to repair. Before joint replacement is selected, moreover, the costs and benefits of alternative procedures should be weighed against the potential for functional restoration with an artificial joint (more will be said about this in later reports).

When defects exist in the stabilizing and moving muscles and their tendons that can be reconstructed only at great cost or to an imperfect degree, joint replacement is indicated only if the "limited goals" approach promises an improvement of function over the preoperative state. This is usually the case with tumors.

If defects in the muscles and tendons (and the bone) cannot be reconstructed, unconstrained replacement is not indicated. Reconstruction with prostheses designed to replace the stabilizing function of the muscles has not yet been adequately tested, although implants for this purpose are available and are undergoing clinical trials.

Individualized solutions are necessary for optimum results in specific cases.

There are definite *contraindications* to replacement arthroplasty, such as radiation damage, immune deficiency (LE), neuroarthropathy (syringomyelia), infection (osteomyelitis, Tuberculosis), compensation claims, and psychiatric disorders.

Besides shoulders which contain so little substance that nothing more can really be done, there are patients who cannot be expected to cope successfully with the demands of reconstruction and rehabilitation.

Finally, the surgeon's appreciation of his own limitations should be a factor in the decision whether or not to undertake prosthetic replacement.

It is consistent with ethical behavior and the Hippocratic oath for the physician to resist external as well as internal pressure in such cases, withhold joint replacement, and thus avoid a course of action that could bring discredit upon the medical profession.

## References

1. Neer CS II, Watson KC, Stanton FJ (1982) Recent experience in total shoulder joint replacement. J Bone Joint Surg [Am] 64: 319-337
2. Post M, Haskell SS, Jablon M (1980) Total shoulder replacement with a constrained prosthesis. J Bone Joint Surg [Am] 62: 327-355

# Technique

# Total Shoulder Replacement - Operative Technique, Postoperative Care, and Functional Assessment

R. P. Welsh and C. R. Constant

Regardless of the type of prosthesis to be implanted in the shoulder, certain principles must be observed if optimum results are to be achieved.

Indeed, total shoulder replacement should be regarded in most instances not as a replacement of the shoulder joint but rather as a rebuilding of the soft-tissue support and a resurfacing of the damaged joint surfaces. This reconstitution of the articular surfaces coupled with rebuilding of the soft tissue of the cuff and muscle support system enables a full rehabilitation of joint function.

Total shoulder replacement, then, should be seen as an essential adjunct to the soft tissue repair, rather than as an end in itself.

The objectives of total shoulder replacement are threefold:

1) resurface the damaged articular structures,
2) rebuild the soft tissue support,
3) rehabilitate shoulder function.

Regardless of the type of device to be implanted, these objectives must be constantly borne in mind. If the joint structure is not rebuilt, the soft tissue repair will be ineffective and rehabilitation efforts negated.

The prosthesis I have chosen to employ over the past nine years is that of Dr. Neer, and I will amplify my comments with regard to the use of this device. I must emphasize, though, that the principles of implantation and management remain the same whatever technical procedure is used.

All techniques involve the following component aspects:

- the surgical approach
- definition of soft-tissue planes
- definition of cuff structure
- resection of the humerus
- preparation of the glenoid
- mobilization of soft-tissue structures
- implantation of the glenoid component
- implantation of the humeral component
- reconstruction of the cuff and soft-tissue support
- closure.

## The Surgical Approach

Above all else in making the surgical approach, the sanctity of the deltoid muscle and axillary nerve must be preserved.

A deltopectoral approach is extended proximally to enable minimal release of the clavicular head of the deltoid if necessary in very muscular individuals. Distally, a partial release of the pectoralis major tendon may further facilitate the exposure.

Shoulder Replacement
Eds.: Kölbel/Helbig/Blauth

## Definition of Soft-Tissue Planes

Careful clearance of the subacromial bursa exposes the rotator cuff tendon. In osteoarthritis or posttraumatic arthritis, the rotator cuff is generally intact. In rheumatoid arthritis, however, 30%-40% of cuffs are torn, and careful debridement of the bursa, synovium, and degenerate tendon is required.

Following clearance of the subacromial space, the subdeltoid space must be defined to separate the deltoid from the tuberosity area to which it may have become adherent. Great care is taken at this stage to protect the circumflex nerve both during dissection and with retraction.

Anterior acromioplasty with complete resection of the coracoacromial ligament will often be necessary, particularly if acromial osteophytes and mechanical impingement are noted. Resection of the lateral articular end of the clavicle at the AC joint should be practiced if this joint is severely involved by the arthritic process.

In both these procedures, great care must be taken to preserve the integrity of the deltoid and its attachments and to keep the posterior AC ligament intact to prevent postoperative AC joint instability.

## Definition of Cuff Structure

Definition of the cuff should be clearly established at this stage, assessing the integrity of the supra- and infraspinatus and defining the subscapularis before further approach is made. In particular, identification of the rotator interval is essential. The subscapularis is now separated from its attachment to the lesser tuberosity, leaving sufficient tendinous material for later reinsertion. As the subscapularis is folded open, the underlying capsule is cleared, and redundant capsule, synovium, and granulation tissue are excised to afford definitive exposure of the humeral head.

## Resection of the Humerus

As in all reconstructive procedures, optimum bone stock must be preserved. The humeral head should be trimmed using a trial prosthesis as a guide to the plane of inclination and retroversion. The arm should be held in 30° of external rotation while this step is done, and the bone carefully resected to preserve the tuberosity insertion of the rotator cuff. The head of the humeral component must extend slightly above the level of the greater tuberosity to prevent impingement of the tuberosity against the acromion during abduction.

With excision of the head, clearance of further capsular and granulation debris is possible, and osteophytes, which can cause substantial anatomic distortion, especially in posttraumatic arthritis, are resected. Any loose bodies should also be removed at this time.

## Preparation of the Glenoid

Essential to an adequate preparation of the glenoid is a clear definition of its margins, particularly anteriorly and inferiorly. Capsular tissue must be cleared and the inferior recess of the shoulder mobilized. It is at this point that the axillary nerve must be carefully protected from injury.

The glenoid margins having been defined, the disposition of the joint face and the integrity of the bony support can be assessed. The glenoid may occasionally require trimming of the joint face with a saw or may even require bone grafting if the margins of support are deficient. In this case a portion of the resected humerus can be used as a graft.

Locating the center of the glenoid and the cancellous cavity can be quite difficult due to distortion of the glenoid by arthritic disease. A notch is prepared initially with a drill point and enlarged sufficiently to allow probing with a curette to define the cancellous space. Care should be taken to avoid penetration of the cortex either anteriorly or posteriorly. With the cavity adequately prepared, a trial implantation of the glenoid is made to ensure a correct disposition of the prosthesis. With the Neer prosthesis, it is preferable to have the glenoid component inclined about 10° with respect to the vertical to provide coverage superiorly, and to set it slightly open-faced to receive the humerus; i. e., the glenoid is anteverted while the humeral head is retroverted.

## Preparation of the Humerus

Probing the medullary canal of the humerus is easy, but care must be taken to set the prosthesis as vertically as possible to avoid the tendency to varus implantation. The humeral head should be trimmed to avoid any bony overhang and provide congruent support for the prosthesis. The humeral prosthesis is selected according to two criteria:

1) the condition of the proximal humerus, which determines the stem size and length, and
2) the available joint space, which determines the head size.

When inserting the humeral prosthesis, there are two vital considerations to be observed: First, it is essential to restore the fulcrum for optimum soft-tissue function. This involves reattachment of the cuff and setting of the deltoid. If the humerus were to be shortened excessively, the function of the deltoid would be compromised, and optimum functional recovery would not be achieved.

In placing the head prosthesis, allowance must be made for the fact that the plane of the scapula is angled 30° to the coronal plane of the body. Thus, the humeral component must be set in 30° of retroversion. This is best achieved by externally rotating the arm 30° and setting the prosthesis square to the coronal axis of the body.

A trial placement of both components can now be made prior to the soft-tissue repair and cementing of the prosthesis.

## Soft-Tissue Repair

With all the bone requirements and the setting for the prosthesis established, the all-important soft-tissue reconstruction can be carried out.

Even if the rotator cuff is intact, the cuff must be separated from the posterior glenoid rim to allow free gliding. This is vital if the cuff is torn, for this at least allows advancement of the cuff to permit reimplantation of the normal insertion to the tuberosity.

Likewise, the subscapularis must be fully mobilized anteriorly so that there will be no interference with its gliding or with external rotation of the shoulder.

Only after the complete soft-tissue support has been drawn together in this manner should the prosthetic components be cemented in place.

## Cementing the Glenoid Component

The glenoid component is cemented first. It is essential to dry the bed thoroughly before implanting the prosthesis. We do this by plugging the glenoid cavity with cement, allowing it to set partially, and then quickly scraping the it of the cavity. At this point the bleeding will be found to be well tamponaded. A new cement plug is then applied, and the prosthesis is implanted definitively. Steady pressure is maintained until the cement hardens.

## Cementing the Humeral Component

The medullary cavity of the humerus is cleared of blood and a cement restrictor placed to prevent distal migration of the cement. A syringe is employed to ensure adequate pressurization, and the implantation is made. Correct positioning of the component is critical. Maintenance of the joint space and a correct retroversion of 25°-40° is essential until the cement is hard. Excessive pressure should be avoided, especially in osteoporotic bone, as it may cause oozing of the cement from the bone.

## Cuff Reconstruction

The rotator cuff is reconstituted and the subscapularis restored, closing the soft-tissue envelope about the shoulder. It should be possible to rebuild the cuff and to allow the arm to rest at full internal rotation. The subscapularis should be reconstituted to allow 30° of external rotation at the time of closure.

Before closing, the shoulder must be put through a range of passive motion to test the strength of the suture lines and the stability of the joint.

## Closure

Formal closure at this stage is simple. The wound is irrigated, a drain inserted, and the subcutaneous tissues and skin are closed. It is rarely necessary to apply a suture to close the deltopectoral interval.

## Postoperative Care

An abduction pillow splint is applied in the operating room with the arm suspended in an overhead sling.

The patient is allowed to mobilize the day after surgery with the arm supported on a 60° abduction wedge.

Pendulum exercises are started the day following surgery, with regular 5-6 times daily workouts of about 5 minutes' duration.

Active assisted exercises with emphasis on flexion, extension, external rotation, and internal rotation are commenced three days after surgery if the cuff is intact. If the cuff has been reconstructed, these exercises are delayed three weeks. Active internal rotation and resisted internal rotation should be delayed two and four weeks, respectively, to allow time for subscapularis healing.

In the hospital it is possible to support the upper extremity with a system of slings and springs which gives active support and allows a degree of passive motion on a continuing basis.

Continuous passive motion has been prescribed on occasion, but its value has yet to be established.

The most important aspect of any therapy program is to recognize that fatiguability will nullify any benefits that are gained. Thus, frequent sessions of short duration and of an intensity below the pain threshold will yield the best results. A hot shower or heat lamp is helpful if applied before the first daily exercise session.

The first four weeks of the rehabilitation program are spent in mobilizing the shoulder. The second four weeks are for strengthening with resistance exercises, although isometric strengthening may be initiated in the third week. From the fourth week on, resistance strengthening is increased as the duration and intensity of effort are gradually improved.

At eight weeks the emphasis is on passive stretching to remove any residual tightness and regain an optimum range of motion.

Thereafter a basic exercise routine should be maintained in all individuals who have undergone a shoulder replacement arthroplasty. Indeed, I would consider that the inability of an individual to participate in a postoperative therapy program and to sustain an ongoing exercise program on an indefinite basis is a contraindication to shoulder replacement. Manipulation should never be necessary with proper technique and aggressive rehabilitation.

## Evaluation of Clinical Results

At this time I shall not specifically refer to the results of total shoulder replacement per se, but would prefer to make some broad comments regarding the evaluation of shoulder function and the results of shoulder surgery in particular.

In whatever we do, it is vital that we be able to quantitate our results so that we can measurably assess the benefits gained or problems persisting.

We should recognize at the outset that in undertaking shoulder replacement surgery, we are attempting to salvage a situation in which the patient's overall function is severely compromised. Often the pain is overwhelming and motion grossly restricted.

It is possible, therefore, to improve the patient's overall status considerably by surgical intervention. But where does such a result lie in relation to that which is "normal" for a subject of the same age without shoulder problems? We must recognize that a deterioration of shoulder function is a natural consequence of aging, and the function that is normal for a 30-year-old may be quite impossible for a normal 70-year-old. Hence, we must express our clinical results in terms of that which might reasonably be expected in a normal individual of the same age.

**Table 1.** Scoring for Individual Parameters

| | |
|---|---|
| Pain | 15 |
| Activities of daily living | 20 |
| Range of motion | 40 |
| Power | 25 |
| Total | 100 |

**Table 2.** Scoring for Pain

| | |
|---|---|
| None | 15 |
| Mild | 10 |
| Moderate | 5 |
| Severe | 0 |

**Table 3.** Scoring for Activities of Daily Living

| | | |
|---|---|---|
| A Activity level: | - Full work | 4 |
| | - Full recreation/sport | 4 |
| | - Unaffected sleep | 2 |
| B Positioning: | - Up to waist | 2 |
| | - Up to xiphoid | 4 |
| | - Up to neck | 6 |
| | - Up to top of head | 8 |
| | - Above head | 10 |
| Total | | 20 |

**Table 4.** Scoring for Forward and Lateral Elevation

| | |
|---|---|
| 0° - 30° | 0 |
| 31° - 60° | 2 |
| 61° - 90° | 4 |
| 91° - 120° | 6 |
| 120° - 150° | 8 |
| 150° - 180° | 10 |

## A System of Functional Assessment

The system we have chosen employs a 100 point score made up of several different parameters (Table 1).

The degree of pain experienced and the ability to perform the normal tasks of daily living are rated subjectively, while the active range of motion and power are objectively measured. In all cases it is essential to record the preand postoperative scores as well as document the performance of the contralateral extremity.

*Pain.* Pain is allocated 15 of the total 100 points, with the absence of pain scoring 15 and severe pain 0. Pain is assessed during the normal daily activities of work, recreation, rest, and sleep (Table 2).

*Activities of daily living.* The subjective ability to perform all activities in which the patient wishes to engage scores 20 points. This includes 10 points for full work, recreational, and sleep activities and 10 points for the ability to move the hand from below the waist to an overhead position (Table 3).

*Range of motion.* The active range of motion achieved is of prime significance in practical terms. This must be determined objectively, and a goniometer should be used to measure the angle of maximum active painless or comfortable motion on the planes of forward and lateral elevation, external rotation, and internal rotation. It should be noted that external rotation implies an associated capability in flexion and abduction, while internal rotaton implies an ability to extend the shoulder (Tables 4–6).

**Table 5.** Scoring for External Rotation

| | |
|---|---|
| Hand behind head with elbow held forward | 2 |
| Hand behind head with elbow held back | 2 |
| Hand on top of head with elbow held forward | 2 |
| Hand on top of head with elbow held back | 2 |
| Full elevation from top of head | 2 |
| Total | 10 |

**Table 6.** Scoring for Internal Rotation

| | |
|---|---|
| Dorsum of hand to lateral thigh | 0 |
| Dorsum of hand to buttock | 2 |
| Dorsum of hand to lumbosacral junction | 4 |
| Dorsum of hand to waist (3rd lumbar vertebra) | 6 |
| Dorsum of hand to 12th dorsal vertebra | 8 |
| Dorsum of hand to interscapular region (7th d.v.) | 10 |

**Table 7.** Shoulder Function

| | Right (score) | Left (score) |
|---|---|---|
| Pain: | | |
| Daily activities: | | |
| - Work | | |
| - Recreation | | |
| - Sleep | | |
| - Position | | |
| Range of motion: | | |
| - Abduction | | |
| - Flexion | | |
| - Int. rotation | | |
| - Ext. rotation | | |
| Power (in lbs.): | | |
| Total | % | % |

*Power*. Power is measured with a simple tensiometer, a spring balance that records the power of shoulder abduction at 90° in pounds. A handle attachment makes the procedure relatively simple even for those with hand deformity, such as rheumatoid arthritics. Patients who do not have 90° of active abduction also can be tested with this method.

Of course this technique is not as accurate as the Cybex II, but it does provide a consistent reflection of shoulder power that is reproducible.

It is important to note that this parameter of measurement is particularly sensitive to a decline of function with age, and bilateral assessments must be routinely undertaken in order to permit a fair comparison.

*Reliability of recording*. These simple techniques have been tested using different observers measuring 100 abnormal shoulders. The observer variance averaged only 3%, indicating a very acceptable degree of reliability.

## Discussion

Recording the results in this way enables a valid comparison to be made between patients of different ages, with different pathologies, and who have undergone different surgical procedures. It brings objectivity to the presentation of results, especially when appropriate preoperative, postoperative, and contralateral assessments are made (Table 7).

## Conclusion

An effort has been made to present the principles of shoulder reconstruction by total shoulder replacement arthroplasty.

It is emphasized that the implantation of a prosthetic device is basically an adjunct to the complete soft-tissue reconstruction and rehabilitation of a severely compromised joint by restoration of the articular surfaces.

Good results can be achieved only by careful attention to detail and a well-supervised postoperative course of rehabilitative therpy.

In recording results, we must endeavor to be as objective as possible and quantitate details of the examination both pre- and postoperatively wherever possible.

If the procedure is performed correctly, its results are good enough to commend it as a procedure of elective reconstruction rather than just a salvage operation for hopeless cases.

## Discussion

*Chairman:* Dr. Welsh, what is your technique for inserting the glenoid component? How can you be sure that you are drilling within the scapular neck and are not penetrating the posterior cortex?

*Welsh:* By clearly defining the margins of the glenoid posteriorly, anteriorly, superiorly, and inferiorly. Only then can I be sure that I am directing the drill bit properly when notching the hard subchondral bone of the glenoid. It is easy to be misled by a posterior osteophyte. First I drill through the subchondral cortex only, then I use a curette to open the space in the scapular neck. This phase is technically very demanding.

*Chairman:* You have shown that you isolate the subscapularis from the capsule before you open the joint. Later you said that you mobilize the subscapularis still farther past the glenoid rim. You did not mention what you do with the capsule.

*Welsh:* Lately I have made it a practice to remove most of the capsule. When I do this, I find that my results are better than when I leave the capsule alone. I believe that I create better conditions for the arthroplasty by clearly defining the rotator cuff, detaching it from the glenoid rim, and removing parts of the capsule that might interfere with motion. I make sure that the subscapularis is dissected free.

*Chairman:* Isn't the anterior capsule necessary for anterior stability?

*Welsh:* I do not believe that the capsule really contributes to shoulder stability after the arthroplasty has been completed. The subscapularis has to be reattached, however. Both of them cannot be removed. I place great importance on mobilizing the subscapularis and reattaching it in such a way that it stabilizes the shoulder anteriorly.

What does Dr. Cofield do with the capsule?

*Cofield:* I do not think one needs to do anything special with the capsule if it is normal. If it is too thick, it should be trimmed to a more normal thickness and flexibility. And if it is too short mediolaterally, it can be released on one side. This will give more length, just as if the capsule were excised. But I do not think that is necessary, and I believe it is enough to remove excess tissue.

*Pahle:* I want to underscore what you said concerning complete visualization of the glenoid. I find the old Bankart retractor very useful for this purpose. When the head has been excised, the Bankart can be passed behind the posterior glenoid rim to the scapular neck to give complete exposure of the glenoid. I would also point out that it is necessary not just to separate the subscapularis from the anterior margin, but also to make sure that an elastic resistance is felt when the muscle is pulled on. This will confirm that the subscapularis can contract effectively; otherwise there is no point is reattaching it.

*Welsh:* I agree completely with both comments. I personally use two narrow Hohmann retractors. The Bankart instrument is excellent, and the Fukuda retractor also can be used.

I did not learn about mobilization of the subscapularis in my initial visit with Dr. Neer. It was only three years later, in a reoperation on one of my patients, that Dr. Neer showed me how extensively he mobilized the subscapularis. The maneuver gave a clear view of the brachial plexus and axillary vessels. I concluded that he obtains a good range of motion postoperatively only when he mobilizes the subscapularis to that extent. Naturally the wide dissection enchroaches somewhat on the axillary nerve, which is dangerously close.

With regard to the cephalic vein, I am in favor of protecting and preserving it if at all possible.

*Laumann:* When the shoulder joint is severely contracted, I feel that the coracohumeral ligament should be resected. I believe that it interferes with mobility after the arthroplasty, and that it should be detached proximally at the superior glenoid margin and at the base of the coracoid process.

What do you do with the long biceps tendon when it is badly damaged? Do you resect it, or do you routinely leave it alone? Or do you leave it only when you have a rotator cuff that you cannot reconstruct?

*Welsh:* Concerning the coracohumeral ligament, I agree that it hampers repair of the rotator cuff in many cases. The same applies to total joint replacement. The ligament should be resected. The subcoracoid space is a gliding space, as are the subacromial and subdeltoid spaces. They must be cleared sufficiently to allow tendon gliding, and that implies resection of the coracohumeral ligament.

As for the biceps, I always try to preserve the tendon of its long head. If the tendon is already attenuated and frayed, I handle it very carefully and leave it alone. I should add that I have seen a later rupture of the long biceps tendon in 3 or 4 of my patients. Perhaps I should have resected the frayed intraarticular portions initially and refixed the tendon to the sulcus.

*Cofield:* Concerning the cephalic vein, it is worth remembering that there is an infraclavicular triangle that is analogous to the femoral triangle. If the dissection is continued proximally beneath the calvicle, it is possible to retract the medial border of the deltoid laterally, leave the vein alone, and ligate only the vessels supplying the deltoid. Then the vein should present no problems. If it does, then it matters very little whether it is ligated primarily or sutured because of injury. I prefer a vascular suture, because I find it easier and safer than a ligature.

In my opinion the coracohumeral ligament is already severed at the time of the arthrotomy - at least it is when I do it. The third point related to the biceps tendon: Ignore it unless it is more than 50% destroyed or no longer firm.

The tendon should not be ignored in rheumatoid arthritis, because it can cause severe complaints if synovitis persists around the biceps tendon in the sulcus. Therefore we routinely open the biceps tendon groove and perform a synovectomy and tenosynovectomy there. If the tendon is torn, as is often the case, the distal stump will usually be adherent to the bone. Then one can use the intraarticular part for reconstructing the damaged rotator cuff. Especially if this part of the tendon is still intact and has good width, it can be used to close the gap between the supraspinatus and infraspinatus. This is a very elegant type of reconstruction.

*Pahle:* You also resect the glenoid labrum. It has an important function in the normal shoulder, that of preventing dislocation. How many dislocations have you seen with your prostheses? Initially I had problems with several dislocations in my own series.

*Welsh:* Well, of course, the glenoid component must be solidly attached, and I make certain that the back of the component is in contact with the bone. I have no use for soft tissues that might come between the implant and the glenoid bone during cementing, and so I resect those tissues.

The importance of the labrum in the normal shoulder joint is well established. But here we are not dealing with a normal situation. The dislocation of a prosthesis would reflect on its stability. The only case in my series of 56 patients with total shoulder implants occurred in a man who had a bone defect of the humerus. In that case I had not restored the length of the humerus, and the prosthesis dislocated inferiorly. Anterior dislocation is not very common. It is possible, but it does not seem to be a problem.

If we want to analyze the dislocation cases, we should 1) recall the preoperative pathologic status of the joint, 2) critically review the individual steps of the operation, and 3) speculate about the past and current status of the reconstructed soft tissues. It is my impression that dislocations result from failure of the soft tissues or from incorrect positioning of the prosthesis.

*Chairman:* How important is the correct degree of retroversion of the humeral component for the stability of the prosthesis?

*Welsh:* I doubt that it is as important as I once believed. While I was with Dr. Neer, I saw that he set the component in 30° to 60° of retroversion, depending on the circumstances. One always has to improvise somewhat according to the situation. A glenoid may be very badly worn anteriorly and may have extensive posterior osteophytes. In this case the glenoid component would have to be set somewhat differently, which in turn would affect the positioning of the humeral component.

We must go by what we find, and our reconstruction cannot always be anatomically perfect. I believe that the range for positioning of the humeral implant is greater than just 30° of retroversion, although that seems to be by far the most frequent position, and probably the most favorable.

*Blauth:* On the subject of assessing results: How much time do you take to fill out your examination form?

*Welsh:* The assistant who works with me and who drew up the form takes about 15 min to examine the subject and complete the form. That is about the right amount of time needed for documentation.

*Blauth:* Is it really worthwhile to perform function tests in a rheumatoid patient? The results are bound to be influenced by the involvement of neighboring joints; and while such a scoring system may be useful in comparing pre- and postoperative status, it is practically useless in other respects. Dr. Pahle shares this opinion. I would like to ask you how many of your patients have rheumatoid disease, and how many of these have multiple disabilities with involvement of only one shoulder?

*Welsh:* I work in a hospital for orthopedic and rheumatic diseases. I perform about 900 operations a year, more than 250 of them in rheumatoid patients; so I have extensive experience with rheumatoid arthritis. Therefore I believe that our scoring system is practical and generally applicable.

Incidentally, we examined a series of patients without rheumatoid arthritis and compared their normal shoulders with the diseased shoulders. The difficulty occurs in rheumatoid patients where there is a need to compare a bad left shoulder with a bad right shoulder. Nevertheless, he have data that tell us what the result in a rheumatoid shoulder would be if we were to compare it with a normal shoulder in an age-matched group. We are trying here to bring objectivity into an area where there is a great tendency to be subjective. Rheumatoid patients are relieved of their pain, and they feel better. They no longer complain, and therefore the result is good. The success rate with this kind of assessment would be 100%. We are trying to be more objective, and we have made some effort to weight the numbers for an overall result. We intend to publish our scoring system in the near future, and it is also treated in the present volume.

Often surgeons are tempted to say that their main objective in performing an operation is to relieve pain. But we also take a look at functional gain, which can radically change the way the rheumatoid patient leads his life. Pain is certainly important, but we have tended to place less emphasis on pain relief, even though it is usually the main criterion for patient selection. It is our intention to quantify the functional gain that is obtained.

# Long-Term Results

# Results of Hemiarthroplasty and Total Shoulder Replacement

R. H. Cofield

Early in the 1970s it was thought that rotator cuff disease would parallel and be proportional to the degree of intraarticular cartilage disease in patients requiring shoulder replacement surgery. In line with this thought, in the early 1970s we used the Bickel and the Stanmore implants, anticipating significant rotator cuff disease. In 1975 we reviewed our experience with these implants and made two observations:

1. Tears of the rotator cuff were much less frequent than we expected.
2. Reoperations with these implants were common, approaching 50% with very short follow-up.

This led us to consider the unconstrained implant, and the most widely recognized one was that designed by Neer with multiple humeral components and now a polyethylene glenoid component [2].

In the late 1970s we analyzed the rotator cuff pathology seen in 176 shoulders that required total replacement arthroplasty. Only 27% had rotator cuff tearing. This lesion was infrequent in osteoarthritis and was seen in approximately one-third of patients with rheumatoid arthritis. In old trauma there was osseous deformity rather than rotator cuff tearing. Those with cuff-tear arthropathy, of course, all had tendon tears. The size of the tendon tears varied considerably, as it does in non-arthritics. Repair of the tendon tears could be accomplished by routine measures in most patients, and so it appeared that over 90% of our patients who required total shoulder replacement could easily be managed with the unconstrained implant.

We performed approximately 500 shoulder replacements between 1975 and 1984. Three major diagnoses were recognized: rheumatoid arthritis, osteoarthritis, and arthritis due to old trauma. Arthritis due to cuff-tear involvement or failed surgery was less common.

## Proximal Humeral Prosthetic Replacement

Proximal humeral surface replacement alone is most commonly used for the treatment of fractures. We have accepted the four-part classification described by Neer, recalling that it is a displacement system. We consider prosthetic replacement in acute injuries for four-part lesions, occasional three-part lesions in elderly patients with severe osteoporosis when a prosthesis would make the fixation much more secure, and of course for those rare head-splitting or impression fractures where more than 40% or 50% of the articular surface is involved. Figure 1 shows an example of a four-part posterior fracture-dislocation treated by a prosthesis. The most serious problem we have seen with these implants in this setting is failure of secure tuberosity fixation and healing of the tuberosities behind the implant. We now use both horizontal and vertical suturing.

For chronic fracture problems, we consider a proximal humeral prosthesis when

Shoulder Replacement
Eds.: Kölbel/Helbig/Blauth

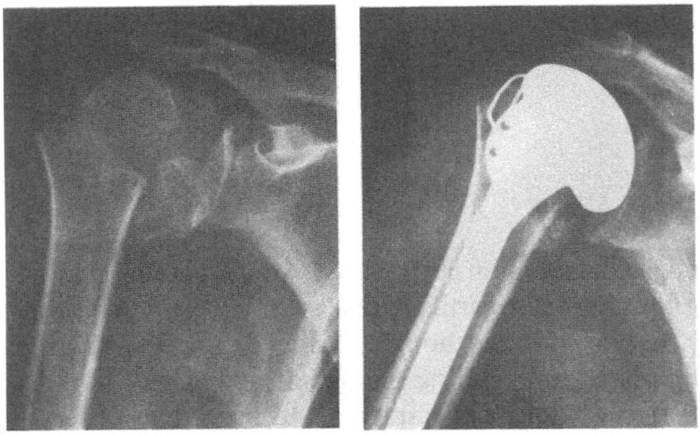

a b

**Fig. 1. a** Man 73 years of age with a 4-part posterior fracture-dislocation. **b** Early postoperative film following insertion of the prosthesis and repositioning and fixation of the greater tuberosity

there is a malunion of the upper humerus with an irregular joint surface, and the glenoid is in reasonably good condition. Hemiarthroplasty is also considered in cases of avascular necrosis and in chronic dislocations when the head fragment is soft, the cartilage has been lost, or there is destruction of more than 50% of the articular surface. Occasionally we consider a prosthesis in a nonunion in an elderly patient when there is a small osteoporotic head fragment. Of course, it may also be considered in lesser degrees of arthritis secondary to many types of injury.

Examples of cases where a prosthesis has been used in chronic traumatic conditions include:

1) an elderly women with a malunion (Fig. 2),
2) a young man with a chronically unreduced posterior fracture-dislocation (Fig. 3),
3) a middle-aged woman with a fracture that went on to avascular necrosis (Fig. 4).

Our series includes 49 patients with fractures who were treated with a prosthesis and followed an average of 3 years (2–10) [3]. In the acute fracture group, pain relief was satisfactory in all patients. In the chronic trauma group, 4 of 31 shoulders did not achieve a satisfactory state regarding pain relief. Postoperative active abduction in the acute fracture group averaged 103° but varied considerably. In the chronic fracture group, postoperative active abduction improved from 64° to 101° and also varied considerably. There were many complications, particularly in the chronic surgery group. These tended to relate both to the difficulty of the surgery and to the difficulty of achieving secure fixation of the tuberosity.

As a result of this experience, we believe that the use of the Neer prosthesis affords satisfactory pain relief in posttraumatic conditions. Motion and strength may be limited. In the acute group this is so because of difficulties with tuberosity fixation, and in the chronic group because of difficulties with tuberosity fixation and scarring. We would advise early surgery in these patients, secure rotator cuff and tuberosity repair, varying the use of external support as needed, and the use of early guided physiotherapy.

In the past we have also tried to avoid using a glenoid component and have used just a proximal humeral replacement in the treatment of rheumatoid arthritis and osteoarthritis. Over a 6-year period, 91 shoulders in 84 patients received this form of treatment. Seventy-eight patients were alive at the time of review, and 72 patients

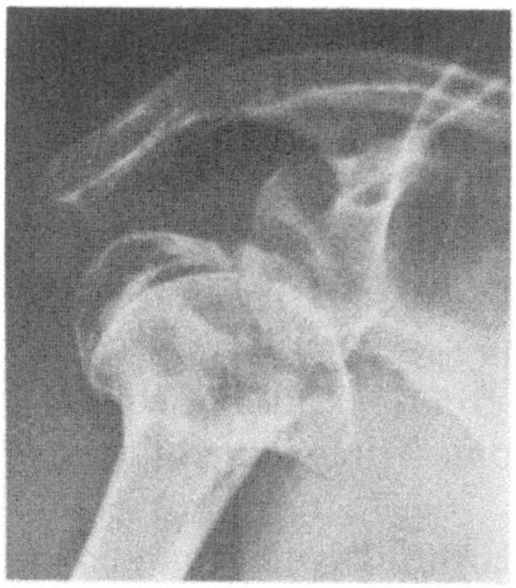

**Fig. 2.** Malunited proximal humeral fracture in an elderly woman

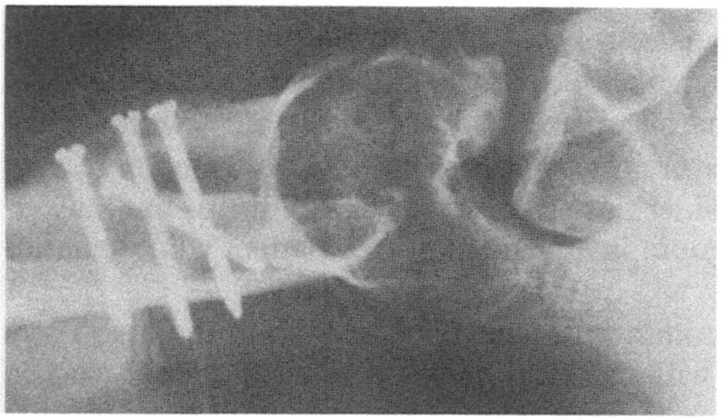

**Fig. 3.** Man 31 years of age was involved in a motorcycle accident and treated elsewhere for delayed union of a humeral shaft fracture. The posterior dislocation with impression of the humeral head was not treated initially

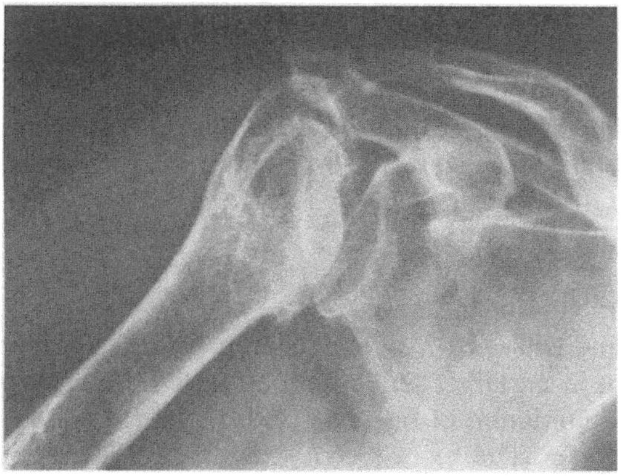

**Fig. 4.** Woman 69 years of age who sustained a comminuted proximal humeral fracture 1½ years earlier. Now there is avascular necrosis of the head fragment with collapse of the bone

with 78 shoulders were available for evaluation at an average of 3 years. Follow-up evaluation ranged from two to six years. A number of adjunctive procedures were necessary in those with rheumatoid arthritis, and as in the larger group, approximately one-third required rotator cuff repair.

Satisfactory pain relief occurred in 88% of those with rheumatoid arthritis but in only 82% of those with osteoarthritis. A number of the latter patients, in fact, had pain relief that would be considered only marginally satisfactory. Return of active movement was less but approached that seen in total shoulder arthroplasties. Patient satisfaction reflected the degree of pain relief, and so the patients with osteoarthritis fared less well in this regard than the patients with rheumatoid arthritis.

Two complications occurred in the rheumatoid patients:
1) brachial plexus paralysis, which resolved, and
2) intraoperative humeral fracture, which was treated by internal fixation at the time of surgery.

Three reoperations were necessary in the rheumatoid group because of continuing pain, and five were necessary in the osteoarthritic group. Three more of the osteoarthritic patients are considering revision.

We concluded from this experience that pain relief in arthritic patients undergoing proximal humeral replacement is not as frequent or as good as with total shoulder arthroplasty. Motion is slightly less than with total shoulder replacement, and failures of the proximal humeral prosthesis occur because of continuing pain. Unfortunately, this problem is unpredictable as far as the individual is concerned. We continue to consider proximal humeral replacement in rheumatoid arthritis when the bone is inadequate, such as in severe osteoporosis or with severe medial resorption of the glenoid. We seldom consider this operation in osteoarthritis but may attempt it when there is only mild glenoid involvement or in a patient who demands heavy use of his arm.

Avascular necrosis is much less common in the shoulder than in the hip. There are a moderate number of patients with avascular necrosis in the shoulder who do not require surgical treatment. When surgery is necessary, the pathology is quite similar to that in the hip, and unless glenoid involvement is pronounced, a proximal humeral prosthesis is used. We have done this in 13 shoulders, and only 1 patient has failed to achieve complete pain relief and more than 80% of normal movement.

## Total Shoulder Replacement

The total shoulder arthroplasty patients were recently reviewed and have been reported in the *Journal of Bone and Joint Surgery* [1]. We limited our analysis to the three major diagnostic categories:
1) rheumatoid arthritis,
2) osteoarthritis,
3) arthritis due to old fractures or fracture-dislocations.

The study group consisted of 65 patients with 73 operated shoulders. The extent of rotator cuff disease paralleled that in the larger series outlined earlier. Follow-up evaluation was by examination at a minimum of one year and by patient contact and X-ray at a minimum of two years. The most recent examination averaged 39 months. The most recent X-ray examination averaged 36 months.

Pain relief occurred in 92% of patients, and return of active motion was 2/3 normal. The range of variation was fairly large but smaller than that seen in the patients with proximal humeral prostheses. Active abduction was most directly related to the extent of rotator-cuff disease, which in turn was related to the diagnosis. When active abduction was less than 90°, there was usually severe progressive rheumatoid arthritis or the presence of a complication. The major complications were rotator-cuff tearing and loosening of the glenoid component. Most reoperations were performed for late glenoid loosening (Fig. 5). One reoperation was done for deltoid

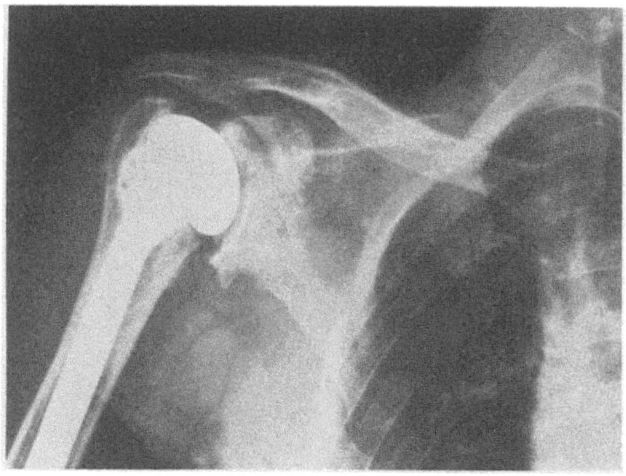

**Fig. 5.** Man 66 years of age who underwent total shoulder arthroplasty 4 years previously. In the last year pain has developed in association with loosening of the glenoid component. Note the medial migration and upward tilting of the component

paralysis and one for evacuation of a hematoma. In addition to the three patients who were reoperated for glenoid loosening, five other patients showed radiographic signs of glenoid loosening. Most patients exhibited lucent lines around the glenoid, and about one-third have lucent lines that continue to be progressive.

Summarizing these results, we feel that unconstrained implants are usually successful, and that, almost without exception, they are the implant of first choice for shoulder replacements at the present time. Prosthetic humeral head replacement continues to have an important role in selected shoulder fractures, in rheumatoid arthritis with glenoid bone loss, and in occasional patients with osteoarthritis. It is also useful in the treatment of avascular necrosis with minimal glenoid surface changes. Total shoulder arthroplasty does relieve pain in approximately 90% of patients, and postoperative motion averages 2/3 normal. However, the results differ from the hip and knee in that there is much variation in the recovery of movement. Failure of total shoulder arthroplasty in our patients is related to late glenoid loosening.

## References

1. Cofield RH (1984) Total shoulder arthroplasty with the Neer prosthesis. J Bone Joint Surg [Am] 66: 899-906
2. Neer CS II, Watson KC, Stanton FJ (1982) Recent experience in total shoulder replacement. J Bone Joint Surg [Am] 64: 319-337
3. Tanner MW, Cofield RH (1983) Prosthetic arthroplasty for fractures and fracture-dislocations of the proximal humerus. Clin Orthop 179: 116-128

# More than Ten Years' Experience with Unconstrained Shoulder Replacement

E. Engelbrecht and K. Heinert

The shoulder joint has been given relatively little attention compared with the joints of the lower extremity. Diseases of the shoulder joint are more readily accessible to treatment by conservative means. Joint-salvaging procedures such as synovectomy, the various types of osteotomy, and resection arthroplasties have specific and limited indications [1]. In the past, *shoulder replacement* has been used only in patients with severe destruction of the bone. Frequently the damage also involves the musculotendinous cuffs and the deltoid, especially after multiple operations. It is common in these cases for severe pain to coexist with irreversible losses of function. The implants that are used in the reconstruction of osteoarthritic shoulders may be one of three types [4]:

1) noninterlocking systems with incongruent articular surfaces (unconstrained type),
2) noninterlocking systems with congruent articular surfaces (semiconstrained type),
3) interlocking prostheses with congruent articular surfaces (constrained type).

The unconstrained and semiconstrained types of prosthesis are most frequently used. In these cases stabilization of the joint by the musculotendinous cuffs and deltoid is as crucial a problem as the need for secure attachment of the glenoid component.

## Prosthetic Systems

Since 1966 we have exclusively used unconstrained prostheses in various combinations. Our earliest operations were hemiarthroplasties using the humeral component of the Neer prosthesis [4, 6]. Later we added a polyethylene glenoid component. In many cases we have used our own model of a spherical humeral head prosthesis (St. Georg model) combined with various types of glenoid cup. As we saw more instances of glenoid loosening, we increasingly returned to the hemiarthroplasty (prosthetic humeral head replacement). We also employ nonprosthetic adjunctive procedures such as osteotomy, deepening of the glenoid cavity, and augmentation of the glenoid roof. We use special tumor prostheses and total humeral prostheses in selected cases (Fig. 1, Table 1).

## Clinical Material and Indications

From 1966 to 1984 we performed a total of 152 prosthetic shoulder operations in 144 patients. Average age at operation was 59 years, with a range from 17 to 81 years. Eight patients underwent bilateral procedures. A sizable percentage of the patients, 22%, had had previous nonprosthetic surgery.

Shoulder Replacement
Eds.: Kölbel/Helbig/Blauth

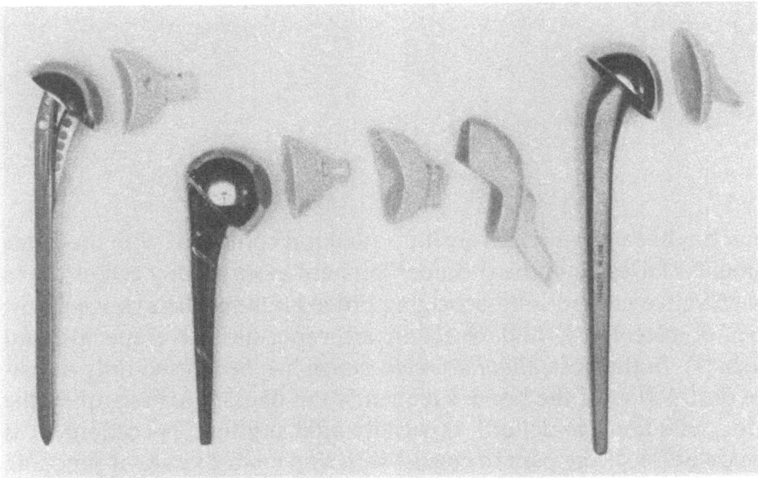

**Fig. 1.** Different types of unconstrained prostheses used from 1966 to 1984

**Table 1.** Types of Unconstrained Shoulder Replacements Used (n = 152)

| | Humeral component | Glenoid component |
|---|---|---|
| 1966-1979 Neer prosthesis | 22 | 8 |
| 1966-1979 St. Georg prosthesis | 41 | 38 |
| 1966-1979 Endo model | 13 | 11 |
| 1966-1979 Partial humeral replacement | 5 | 5 |
| 1966-1979 Total humeral replacement | 1 | 1 |
| 1979-1984 St. Georg prosthesis | 5 | - |
| 1979-1984 Endo model | 59 | - |
| 1979-1984 Partial humeral replacement | 4 | - |
| 1979-1984 Total humeral replacement | 2 | - |

The most frequent indication was posttraumatic arthritis (27%), followed by acute fracture-dislocations in older patients (22%) and idiopathic osteoarthritis (13%). The tumor cases (11%) usually required special prostheses for partial or total humeral replacement. Rare indications were osteoradionecrosis and dysplasia. Eighteen percent of the 152 operations were revisions.

## Operative Technique

Until 1970 we routinely used a standard anterior approach. After finding that division of the anterior and proximal posterior musculotendinous cuffs was often followed by function loss from damage to the capsule and anterior deltoid, since 1978 we have preferred a modification of the Kocher posterior approach for primary implantations [5]. We reserve the anterior approach for special cases such as previously operated shoulders with residual internal fixation material or for tumors that require special prostheses.

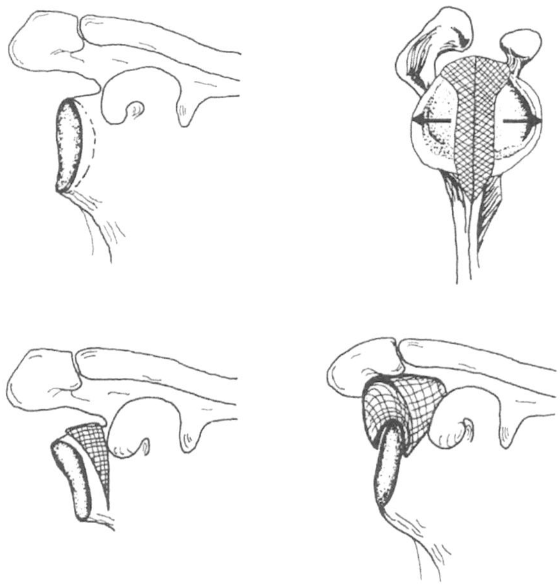

**Fig. 2.** Osteotomies and bone grafts of the glenoid

The patient is operated on in the sitting position. The skin is opened with an S-shaped incision, and the posterior and middle origins of the deltoid are mobilized by osteotomy of the acromion. The proximal posterior musculotendinous cuffs are detached from the greater tuberosity on a small piece of bone. The anterior portion of the capsule and the biceps tendon are left alone. After resection of the head, the humeral prosthesis is cemented into place, setting it in about 20°-30° of retrotorsion to the transverse epicondylar plane. If there is lack of congruity with the glenoid surface, the glenoid cavity is either deepened, osteotomized, wedge-osteotomized, or its roof is augmented with an autologous or homologous cancellous graft (Fig. 2).

Adjunctive procedures to hemiarthroplasty:

- Glenoid osteotomy and cancellous graft 8
- Glenoid roof augmentation 4
- Glenoid deepening 7
- Deltoid transfer 5
- Duraplasty of the capsule 3

The objective of these measures is to buttress the humeral head prosthesis against loads directed superomedially and thereby compensate for any capsuloligamentous deficiency that may exist. The musculotendinous cuffs are reattached with transosseous sutures made of absorbable material. Areas of capsular destruction should be reconstructed, possibly with lyophilized dura [3].

When there is damage to the anterior part of the deltoid, our proximal posterior approach affords an opportunity to transfer intact middle and posterior portions of the deltoid anteriorly. To date we have done transfers of this type in five corrective operations, with satisfying results.

We have performed 45 operations from this approach since 1977. So far we have had no problems with nerve or vascular damage relating to the surgery.

The operative technique and unconstrained prosthesis require that the arm be immobilized postoperatively on an abduction splint for about 6 weeks.

## Clinical Results

Our small series of 152 operations in the last 15 years is too nonhomogeneous to permit a valid statistical evaluation, and standardized methods for the analysis of clinical results still need to be developed in this area.

We were able to follow 51 of the joints operated prior to 1978, with an average follow-up time of more than 4 years. Of the 59 patients who were treated with a humeral head prosthesis since 1979, 35 have been followed an average of 1½ years.

Comparison of the two series showed virtually no differences in terms of *pain relief*: 88% of the patients operated before 1978 (group 1) reported complete or marked pain relief, as opposed to 91% of patients in group 2. Severe residual complaints were attributable to glenoid loosening, dislocation, or trauma-related nerve damage.

Moderate residual complaints, often weather-related, were frequently localized in the anterior capsule or were caused by abnormal tension in the shoulder and neck muscles, especially in cases where shoulder function was restricted. *Joint function* was assessed by measuring the total range of shoulder motion, i.e., by adding together the angular ranges of abduction with and without the scapula, retroversion and elevation, and external and internal rotation. Because of the small case number and the subjectivity of the measurement, we are unable to draw a definitive conclusion. We noted that total shoulder motion in the two groups was restricted preoperatively to 115° and 105°, respectively. After surgery group 1 experienced an average increase of approximately 80°, and group 2 approximately 140°. The greatest increase was noted in joints with rheumatoid disease.

## Complications

Two patients out of 152 (1.3%) developed infections. Both infections occurred prior to 1977.

*Mechanical loosening* is known to be a problem in total shoulder replacements [2]. Our series includes only 1 case of stem loosening; 32 (51%) of the glenoid components became loose.

Complications 1966–1978:

| | |
|---|---|
| Glenoid loosening | 32 (51%) |
| Stem loosening | 1 |
| Early dislocation | 10 |
| Late dislocation | 7 |
| Late subluxation | 7 |
| Ossification | 4 |
| Complications 1979–1984: | |
| Late subluxation | 5 |
| Infection rate 1966–1984: | |
| (n = 152) | |
| Infection | 2 = 1.3% |

The peak incidence of glenoid loosening occurred in the 4th postoperative year, the large Mark II components being affected most frequently (see Fig. 1). Initially we replaced the loose glenoid components with special models, but since 1978 we have made it a practice to remove the loose components entirely. We corrected significant glenoid deficiency by using osteotomy and bone grafting to create a solid, trough-shaped bed to accommodate the humeral component (see Fig. 2). In later years we adopted these corrective procedures for primary replacements of the humeral head alone.

*Dislocations* are a specific complication of unconstrained prostheses. They reflect a deficiency of the musculotendinous cuffs and possibly of the deltoid muscle, as well as inadequate buttressing of the humeral head prosthesis in the glenoid. We can distinguish:
1) early postoperative dislocation anterodistally and
2) slowly progressive subluxation,
which are manifested clinically by poor function and radiographically by migration of the prosthesis toward the roof of the shoulder cavity. With deficiency of the anterior musculotendinous cuffs and the anterior deltoid, late anteroproximal dislocation can occur (Fig. 3).

*Periarticular ossification* was noted in four cases and may account for the limitation of function.

## Discussion

Our experience with shoulder prostheses is based on 126 primary operations and 27 corrective operations performed since 1966. Our indication for prosthetic surgery was a painful joint with impaired function due to various causes.

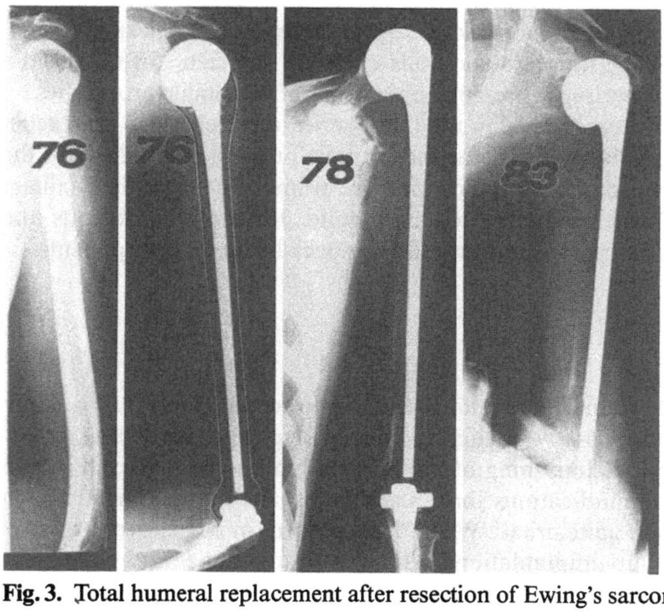


**Fig. 3.** Total humeral replacement after resection of Ewing's sarcoma; late dislocation

We have followed our surgical patients for 10 years or more, but the nonhomogeneity of our clinical material makes it difficult to evaluate our small series, and meaningful statistical conclusions cannot be drawn. Nevertheless, our clinical results and the failures that occurred have enabled us to develop a more rational approach to the prosthetic management of these shoulders.

The high rate of glenoid loosening illustrates the problem of obtaining secure attachment of the glenoid component. Because of this problem, we returned in 1979 to prosthetic replacement of the humeral head only, without replacing the glenoid. At the same time we abandoned the anterior approach in favor of a proximal posterior approach for the reasons stated earlier. Through adjunctive measures on the glenoid cavity (see Fig. 2), we attempt to create a broad abutment for the humeral prosthesis to compensate for capsular insufficiency. If a tumor necessitates partial or complete resection of the musculotendinous cuff, the foregoing measures can be used to prevent late anteroproximal dislocation (see Fig. 3).

We have found the hemiarthroplasty to be as effective as total arthroplasty in alleviating pain, with more than 90% of patients reporting complete or substantial pain relief. The functional results regarding the ability to perform essential movements were not satisfactory in the first series prior to 1978. It appears that the modified operative technique also has a beneficial effect on joint function. The essential factors in this regard are preservation of the anterior capsular and muscular tissues in the posterior approach, fixation of the fulcrum of the humeral prosthesis by buttressing it against a bony trough, and improved techniques in the reconstruction of the musculotendinous cuffs. To date we have observed no proximomedial migration of the prosthesis in the bony bed, and the risk appears small given the relatively non-weight-bearing status of the joint. If problems of this kind arise in the future, one solution might be to line the reconstructed cavity secondarily with a polyethylene shell.

Except for one case, mechanical loosening has involved only the glenoid component. The risk of loosening appears to increase with the degree of congruity between the components. A system with minimal congruity, as illustrated by a shallow glenoid, improves the stability of the anchorage, but it increases the risk of proximal dislocation, especially if the musculotendinous cuffs are deficient. In the last six years we have not had to perform corrective operations after hemiarthroplasties.

Because of our positive experience in the latest series with regard to pain relief and complication rate, we believe that the indications for hemiarthroplasty of the shoulder can be broadened. Contraindications are primary neuropathy, axillary nerve palsy, and significant destruction of the deltoid. Rheumatoid arthritis and neoplasia do not contraindicate hemiarthroplasty, especially in younger patients.

## Summary

Our experience with 126 primary operations and 27 corrective operations in shoulders with prostheses indicates a very high incidence of glenoid loosening, as opposed to virtually no risk of loosening of the humeral component. Except in patients with neuropathy, the indications for replacing only the humeral head (hemiarthroplasty) can be made quite broad. When there is need for corrective surgery of the glenoid, even in primary implantations, adjunctive osteotomies and bone grafting procedures can be used to create a sound abutment for the humeral prosthesis.

The posterior approach with osteotomy of the acromion offers significant advantages over the anterior approach in terms of functional outcome. Our hemiarthroplasty can significantly improve complaints in the severely damaged shoulder, and 90% of patients so treated have been satisfied with the result.

## References

1. Benjamin A (1974) Double osteotomy of the shoulder. Scand J Rheumatol 3: 65
2. Cofield RH (1984) Total shoulder arthroplasty with the Neer prosthesis. J Bone Joint Surg [Am] 66: 899-906
3. Engelbrecht E (1984) Ten years of experience with unconstrained shoulder replacement. In: Bateman JE, Welsh P (eds) Shoulder surgery. Mosby, Toronto London, pp 234-239
4. Engelbrecht E, Siegel A, Röttger J, Heinert K (1980) Erfahrungen mit der Anwendung von Schultergelenksendoprothesen. Chirurg 51: 794-800
5. Kocher T (1902) Excisionen und Resectionen. Obere Extremität. Chirurgische Operationslehre, Bd 4. Fischer, Jena
6. Neer CS, Watson KC, Stanton FJ (1982) Recent experience in total shoulder replacement. J Bone Joint Surg [Am] 64: 319

## Discussion

*Chairman:* Concerning your technique for expanding the glenoid, can you tell us how you perform your longitudinal osteotomy without causing the anterior glenoid rim to break off anteriorly, or the posterior rim to break off posteriorly.

*Engelbrecht:* Your question is certainly justified. That has happened in a few cases, but afterward we have found that another bony bed forms for the prosthesis, and that it consolidates without fixation. Of course you should have an optimum repair of the musculotendinous cuffs, if they are intact, because that will give stability to the whole joint.

*Chairman:* Will you continue to release the deltoid in your approach, even though an approach is now available that no longer requires this?

*Engelbrecht:* At the present time I would say yes. It may be that we can use a somewhat smaller incision than the very extensive one we now employ. This is something we need to learn more about. We need to take into account the experience of Dr. Cofield and see whether we might perhaps get better results with the anterior approach he has described.

*Chairman:* You are referring to the long deltopectoral approach that Neer uses in his technique.

*Hipp:* You have shown some very extensive glenoid roof plasties. I have some difficulties with them, because according to my understanding of anatomy, they would seriously violate the muscles around the glenoid.

*Engelbrecht:* In cases where we have done these procedures, it has been necessary to sacrifice the supraspinatus. You have to resect that muscle and also freshen the inferior aspect of the acromion and the upper portions of the neck of the glenoid roof and the glenoid if possible so that a bone block can be attached there. We attach the block with a small screw inserted through the acromion.

*Helbig:* What problems have you had with the axillary nerve during posterior release of the deltoid?

*Engelbrecht:* To date we have not seen any axillary nerve damage at all, and I hope that will continue to be the case. This may be due to the fact that we release the entire posterior part, so that the whole muscle falls downward and forward and offers protection for the nerve. Clinically we have seen some atrophy of the posterior part of the deltoid, but so far this has had no adverse effects on function. Experience teaches us, I believe, that the anterior structures are by far the most important, and these can be spared by using a posterior approach.

*Tillmann:* One question on the prosthesis that is no longer used today: The glenoid components that had an extended rim, and which performed a function that is now assumed by the reconstructed glenoid roof - did these components have a greater tendency to loosen than the units without special rims?

*Engelbrecht:* Most definitely. We can say with great certainty that the greater the congruity between the head and socket, the greater the tendency toward glenoid loosening. The earliest and most frequent loosenings occurred with the St. Georg Mark II prostheses. So far we have not seen this problem with the shallow cups of the latest generation, although we have seen dislocations.

*Chairman:* That would contradict Dr. Welsh's experience that dislocation is not a real problem. Is that due to the size of the glenoid component?

*Engelbrecht:* I really can't say. Our own experience has been that dislocation is a significant complication.

*Willert:* Concerning subluxations and proximal displacements of your heads: How do you account for this phenomenon, and what can be done about it? Almost all heads migrate superiorly.

*Engelbrecht:* The phenomenon you describe signifies insufficiency of the musculotendinous cuff, and that is why we try increasingly to establish a compensatory buttress on the glenoid side.

*Gottstein:* We have heard much about the importance of soft-tissue reconstruction about the shoulder. When you encountered defects in the rotator cuff, did you resect the cuff and perform a glenoid roof plasty?

*Engelbrecht:* When we were using the anterior approach for arthroplasties, we routinely detached the subscapularis and the supraspinatus, and thus performed a very extensive release of the musculotendinous cuffs. This may have been one reason for our relatively poor results. We tried to reattach these cuffs as accurately as possible with transosseous sutures, but deficiencies still occurred. Generally we immobilized the arm for 6 weeks on an abduction splint to await healing of the reattached musculotendinous cuffs before starting physiotherapy.

*Chairman:* Your series included a number of tumor cases, and thus cases in which you probably would not have been able to reconstruct the rotator cuff even if you had wanted to. Therefore it is very difficult to make valid comparisons.

# Total Shoulder Replacement: Long-Term Results

K.C. Watson

## Evolution

The development of total shoulder replacement in the United States has paralleled that of other joints. Prior to the 1950s, surgery on the shoulder for painful arthritic states was limited to arthrodesis or resection arthroplasty. Debridement was only temporarily and marginally beneficial, and the functional results of arthrodesis or resection left much to be desired. In the early 1950s Dr. Neer began to use a metal humoral prosthesis - a hemiarthroplasty - for certain fractures and milder forms of arthritic degeneration. This prosthesis has proven to be quite durable and effective for these indications, but is was recognized that there were certain conditions with extensive glenoid involvement or bone loss that could not be adequately managed with such a device. A constrained device was an appealing alternative because of the theoretical advantage of providing the stability needed in such instances, and early investigative work was done in this area. The conclusions reached in this early research indicated that a constrained device was not adequately powered when the rotator cuff was sacrified. The loss of function of the infraspinatus and the teres minor as external rotators led to poor functional levels. Conversely, when the muscle power was preserved, fixation of the prosthesis became a problem, or the components would fail. This sequence of events has been experienced by others working in the area of constrained joint replacement. It was concluded that a constrained device invited mechanical failure or was powered inadequately by the deltoid alone, and that such a device was inappropriate in young or active patients and in patients with weak bone. The early enthusiasm for a constrained prosthesis gave way to development of an unconstrained device that would conform more closely to normal anatomy while providing no mechanical linkages to break or transmit excessive forces to the fixation. This approach, however, requires greater attention to the repair and reconstruction of the soft tissues in order to provide stability and restore function.

## The Components

The prosthesis as currently used consists of a metal humeral component (redesigned from the earlier model) that maintains a radius of curvature of 44 mm in two head lengths. The shorter head can be used to facilitate repair of the rotator cuff when it is contracted or deficient. Three different stem sizes are provided to allow for a press-fit in most cases, and several special stems are available for use in unique situations.

The glenoid component is a polyethylene resurfacing device that conforms to the radius of the humeral component. Several designs have been utilized, but the one with the most clinical experience is the 10810. This component has recently been fit-

Shoulder Replacement
Eds.: Kölbel/Helbig/Blauth

ted with a metal backing to prevent cold flow deformation and plastic fatigue at the junction of the keel and the surface. The larger semiconstrained devices were used in a few extremely deficient situations but have not been used in several years because of their fairly high incidence of loosening.

## Technique

The shoulder is approached through a long deltopectoral incision. We preserve the origin of the deltoid, preferring to release some of the deltoid insertion if needed. However, the deltoid often can be retracted quite adequately by abducting the arm. The subscapularis is divided at its insertion on the lesser tuberosity, and the arm is externally rotated to dislocate the humeral head. It is often helpful to remove inferior osteophytes to identify the calcar of the humerus before making the cut to resect the head. Careful attention must be given to maintaining a normal retroversion. The use of a trial humeral component as a guide is helpful. The fin on the component usually sits at the biceps groove between the tuberosities. After the canal is reamed with medullary rasps, a press-fit can be tried. Methylmethacrylate can be used if the fit is not acceptable.

Before final placement of the humeral component, the necessity of resurfacing the glenoid must be assessed. The articular cartilage is often worn unevenly and may appear almost normal in some areas. Often it is worthwhile to probe the cartilage with a needle to determine its thickness. All of the remaining articular cartilage should be removed prior to seating the glenoid component. Once the subchondral bone is exposed, a slot is made in the face of the glenoid to accommodate the keel of the component. Care is taken to avoid penetration of the posterior or anterior cortices. The slot is deepened with a small curette, rather than with a high-speed burr. The trial component must fit flush against the subchondral bone without any rocking or tilting. Any remaining cancellous bone is then curetted out, especially at the base of the coracoid and down the lateral aspect of the scapula, to provide better dispersion of the methylmethacrylate.

A dry field is essential to a good cementing job. After the glenoid is inserted and the cement has dried, the unit is carefully tested for looseness. If there is any indication that a completely tight and congruent fit is not present, the unit is recemented. The humeral component is then implanted and the shoulder reduced. The trial motion at this stage should be smooth and stable. There should be no catching or translation of the prosthesis.

The subscapularis may on occasion, when contracted, require lengthening by Z-plasty, or closure of a scarred and contracted rotator cuff may require use of the short head prosthesis. The deltoid insertion is then repaired if necessary, and a routine skin closure is followed by a standard sling and swathe. An abduction brace may be substituted as circumstances require.

## Indications

The primary objective of total shoulder replacement is pain relief.

Ninety percent of patients seen for total shoulder replacement fall into one of three diagnostic categories:

- Osteoarthritis
- Posttraumatic arthritis
- Rheumatoid arthritis.

Other categories comprising the final 10% include:

- Avascular necrosis
- Revision
- Cuff-tear arthropathy
- Miscellaneous.

## Contraindications

The contraindications also fall into three categories and are similar to those in other joints:

- Infection
- Paralysis
- Neuroarthropathy.

## Results

Overall pain relief has been uniformly good in all categories. Functional recovery is directly related to diagnostic category in that it reflects the status of the soft tissues.

Osteoarthritics and mild rheumatoids have a better overall functional prognosis than patients with posttraumatic arthritis, and the latter tend to have better results than patients undergoing revision surgery or who have massive rotator cuff deficits (e.g., cuff-tear arthropathy, advanced rheumatoid arthritis).

An intensive study of the durability of the glenoid component in 194 total shoulder replacements with an average follow-up of 3 years revealed an identifiable lucent zone at the bone-cement interface in 30% of cases, regardless of the diagnostic category or the patient's level of activity. In most cases these lines were most conspicuous on the axillary view and often were identified on the earliest postoperative films. There were only two cases in which the lucent zone appeared to increase, indicating loosening, and both patients were asymptomatic. Others have reported a higher percentage of lucent lines, but still very few patients have required additional surgery because of loosening. Subsidence or medial migration of the glenoid has occurred in some patients with long-standing osteoporosis (e.g., advanced rheumatoids), and there have been several instances of fracture of the glenoid component at the junction of the face and keel. This has been attributed to inadequate support under the face of the component, subjecting the junction to a rocking or tilting force producing failure from fatigue. Although the number of patients exhibiting this mode of failure so far is quite small, the metal-backed modification was introduced to minimize this complication and is currently preferred in young or active patients. This component, however, is necessarily thicker and may not be accommodated in some small or tight shoulders. Also, in patients with very shallow glenoids it may be necessary to shorten the keel of the glenoid for a flush fit, which cannot be done in the metal-backed unit.

## Rehabilitation

Rehabilitation of the patient with an unconstrained shoulder replacement is more difficult and more essential to the success of the procedure than when a constrained device is used. The goal is pain-free function and as normal a range of motion as possible.

The recovery exercises often must be individualized to protect tenuous rotator cuff repairs or to prevent stress in an unstable position during the healing period. Early motion is ideal and can be accommodated in 80% of cases where there is good cuff repair and adequate stability. The usual regimen calls for passive exercises beginning with the pendulum in the first few postoperative days and progressing to pulley exercises as comfort and stamina permit. External rotation and internal rotation are added as progress is made with the initial exercises.

Active exercises often can be added by the end of the second week, but early emphasis is on obtaining an acceptable passive range. The early application of constant passive motion has shortened the initial phase of rehabilitation in many cases. Patient acceptance and compliance have been quite good.

In contrast to patients in whom early motion is desirable, there are some patients who require bracing (e.g., patients with a tenuous rotator cuff repair and many rheumatoids). Even while in the brace, however, it is often possible to begin exercises which do not jeopardize the repair. After 3-6 weeks the brace is removed, and a modified rehabilitation program is begun depending on the goals that may be expected. In other situations where there has been chronic dislocation, it may be necessary to prevent excessive rotation during the healing process. This may require use of a specially designed brace.

After an acceptable early range of motion has been attained, gentle strengthening exercises are initiated using elastic bands or tubing. These are designed to strengthen the rotator cuff without stressing any repair and may be deferred as the situation demands.

Finally, maintenance exercises are undertaken when there has been maximum improvement. These are usually done once daily to prevent gradual loss of motion and may be continued for years.

## Complications

The complication rate has been quite low considering the condition of many of the patients and the quality of their tissues. They are often older, and many have had previous surgery. Fortunately thromboembolism, which plagues prosthetic surgery in the lower extremities, has not been a problem. Nor has there been the incidence of devastating late hematogenous infection like that which has occurred like a time bomb in lower limb joint replacements. Infection usually occurs as a result of previous contamination in cases with prior surgery, and fortunately it is very rare in patients having their first operation. When an infection develops, of course, the components have to be removed, and the patient is necessarily left with a flail shoulder. There have been a few attempts at converting this situation to an arthrodesis when excessive migration of the proximal humerus is painful, but this procedure is quite difficult.

Most other complications cause a deterioration in function, but often there is still acceptable control of pain, making the necessity of reoperation less frequent than the actual complication rate.

## Discussion

Degenerative, traumatic, and arthritic shoulder problems that involve the glenoid as well as the humeral head can almost all be managed satisfactorily with an unconstrained prosthesis. This approach, while more difficult from a technical standpoint, has the advantage of better durability than any constrained replacement. Significant deficits of bone and muscle can be effectively handled and do not preclude the use of an unconstrained device.

Clinical experience indicates that the results of shoulder replacement surgery are as predictable and effective as those of other joint replacements.

## References

Neer CS, Watson KC, Stanton FI (1982) Recent experience in total shoulder replacement. J Bone Joint Surg [Am] 64: 319-337

# Shoulder Replacement in Rheumatoid Arthritis

# Total Shoulder Replacement in Rheumatoid Arthritis

A. Lettin

The Stanmore total shoulder replacement was introduced into clinical practice in 1969 by Lettin and Scales, although replacement of the humeral head alone for fractures was already well established by that time. Earlier experience at the Royal National Orthopedic Hospital showed that resection and replacement of the upper end of the humerus with a massive prosthesis for tumors was invariably followed by upward and forward subluxation of the prosthesis in the glenoid. This was attributed to the lack of the stabilizing action of the rotator cuff, leaving the upward pull of the deltoid unopposed. This need for a stable fulcrum is also apparent after primary excision of the humeral head when active flexion and abduction of the arm is very limited, although the passive range may be complete (Fig. 1).

These observations led to the design of a constrained ball and socket prosthesis whose components were anchored to the bone with acrylic cement. The small size of the anatomic glenoid and the frail nature of the scapula make fixation of the cup difficult. It cannot be contained within the bone in the way that the acetabular component of a hip replacement is contained by the anatomic acetabulum (Figs. 2 and 3).

In 1982 Lettin, Copeland, and Scales reported the results of 50 Stanmore total shoulder replacements which had been inserted over a period of 10 years with a minimum follow-up of 2 years. One patient died in the early postoperative period, and nine prostheses had to be removed - one for infection, one for recurrent dislocation, and seven for aseptic loosening:

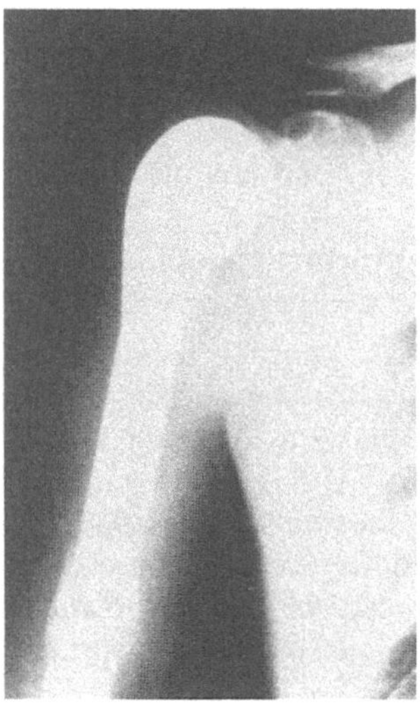

**Fig. 1.** Superior subluxation of a massive replacement for a giant cell tumor

Shoulder Replacement
Eds.: Kölbel/Helbig/Blauth

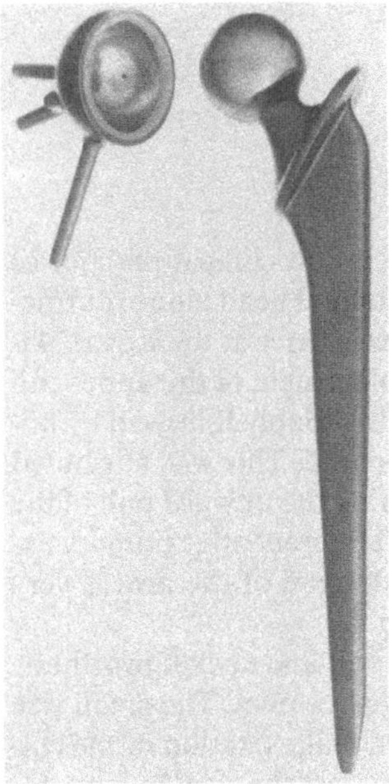

Fig. 2. Stanmore right total shoulder replacement

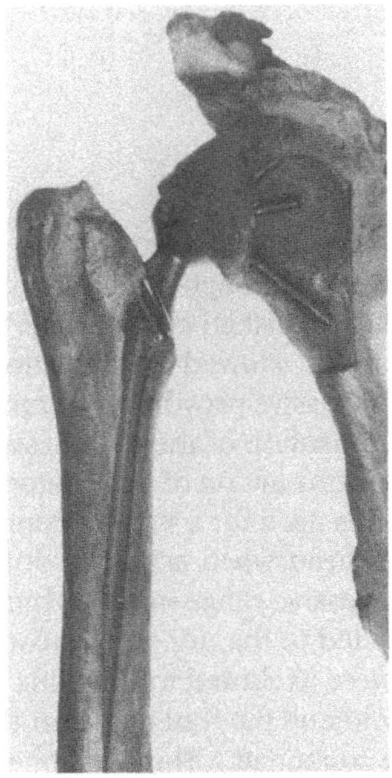

Fig. 3. Technique of fixation of a Stanmore total shoulder replacement

Stanmore total shoulder replacement:
50 Patients 31-81 years of age (average 56.5 years)
 1 Died
 7 Aseptic loosening
 1 Septic loosening
 1 Recurrent dislocation
40 Patients reviewed 2-10 years after replacement.

After the operation most patients were free from pain, and their range of motion had improved. Flexion and abduction improved an average of 20°, but medial rotation improved most dramatically by an average of 40°. This proved to be most significant from a functional standpoint, for most everyday activities are carried out below shoulder level and depend more on medial rotation than any other movement of the shoulder (Table 1, Figs. 4-7).

Although most of the patients were satisfied with their prosthetic shoulder, this is probably a reflection of the severity of their disabilities before operation rather than the excellence of the prosthetic device (Table 2).

Fortunately, when the prosthesis was removed, the resulting excision arthroplasty proved to be more stable than a primary excision arthroplasty, leaving the patient no worse than before the original operation (Table 3, Figs. 8-10).

In 1974 Neer reported the results of humeral head replacement in osteoarthritic patients with the Vitallium prosthesis that previously had been recommended only for the treatment of fractures. In one patient the glenoid also was resurfaced with a polyethylene insert. Since that time this prosthesis has been used extensively in patients suffering from a variety of conditions.

In 1982 Neer, Watson, and Stanton reported the results of 194 replacements using

**Table 1.** Average Gain in Range of Movement with the Stanmore Prosthesis. IR Internal Rotation, ER External Rotation

| | | Flexion | Extension | Abduction | IR | ER |
|---|---|---|---|---|---|---|
| Rheum. arthritis | 66% | | | | | |
| Osteoarthritis | 10% | 20° | 20° | 20° | 40° | 10° |
| Post-trauma | 20% | | | | | |
| Revision | 4% | | | | | |

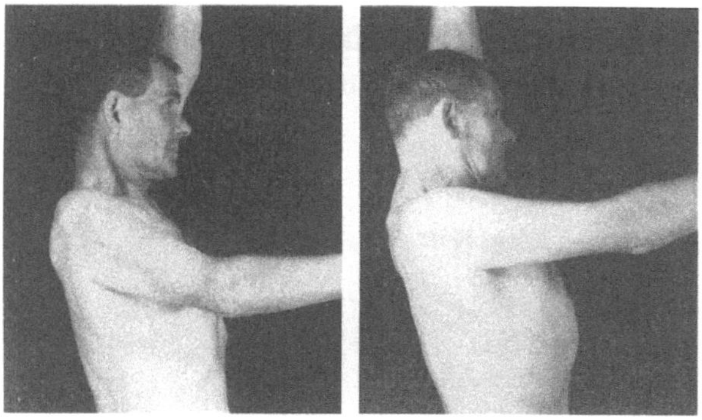

a b

**Fig. 4a,b.** Flexion **a** before and **b** after right total shoulder replacement

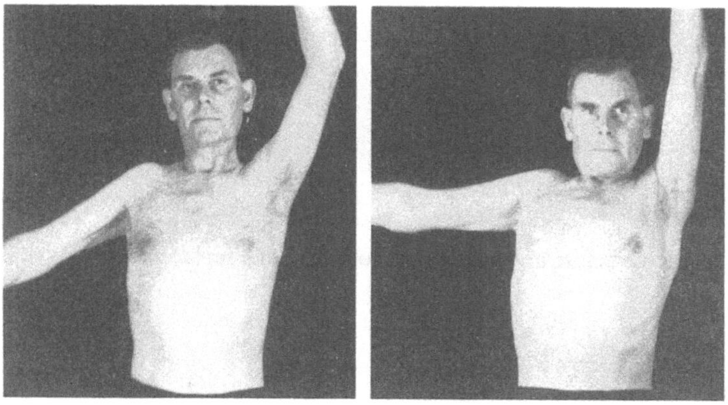

a b

**Fig. 5a,b.** Abduction **a** before and **b** after right total shoulder replacement

this unconstrained resurfacing prosthesis with a minimum follow-up of 2 years and a maximum of 8 years (average 3 years). It is difficult to compare these results with those of the Stanmore prosthesis for a number of reasons. Only 33% of the Neer prostheses were used in patients with rheumatoid arthritis; the authors themselves point out the importance of evaluating results according to diagnostic category, and rheumatoid patients present the greatest difficulty. They also excluded cases from evaluation in which the expectation of success was so low that they were treated on a "limited goals" basis. Seven of the 50 patients with rheumatoid arthritis were in this category. The remaining 43 patients gained an average of 57° of elevation and 60° of external rotation. Unfortunately, no mention is made of internal rotation, which appears to be the most useful functional movement, and there is no indica-

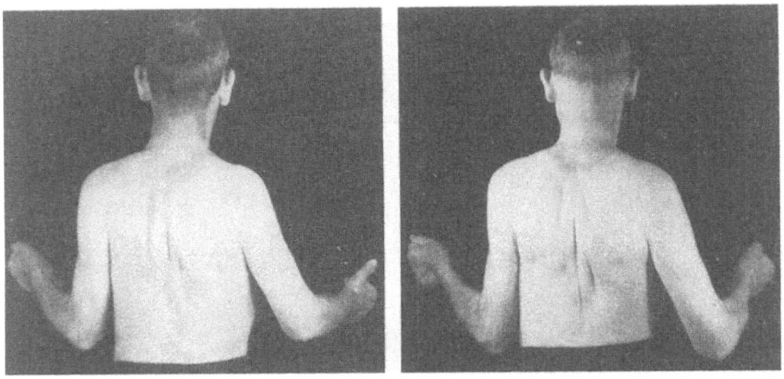

a b

**Fig. 6 a,b.** External rotation **a** before and **b** after right total shoulder replacement

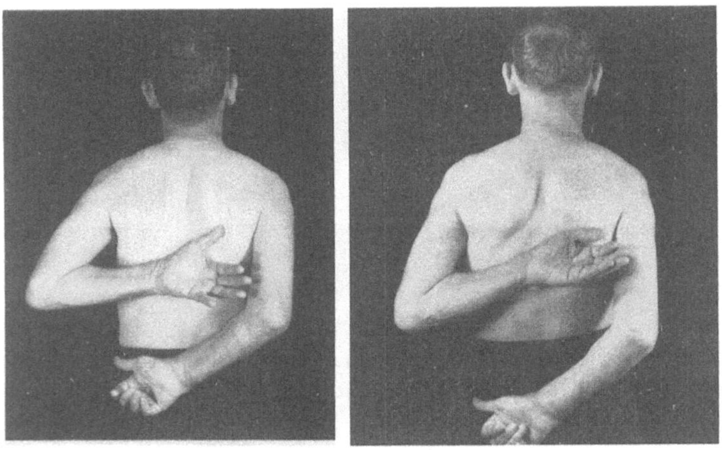

a b

**Fig. 7 a,b.** Internal rotation **a** before and **b** after right total shoulder replacement

**Table 2.** Results of Self-Assessment in 36 Patients

| | Better | Same | Worse |
|---|---|---|---|
| Pain | 32 | 4 | 0 |
| Range of movement | 26 | 9 | 1 |
| Function | 29 | 5 | 2 |

**Table 3.** Results of Self-Assessment in 9 Patients before Replacement and after Removal of the Prosthesis

| | Better | Same | Worse |
|---|---|---|---|
| Pain | 8 | 1 | 0 |
| Range of movement | 4 | 3 | 2 |
| Function | 3 | 3 | 3 |

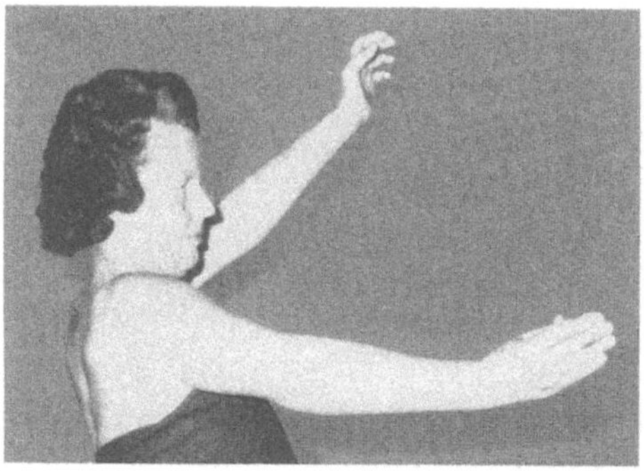

**Fig. 8.** Flexion after removal of right total shoulder replacement

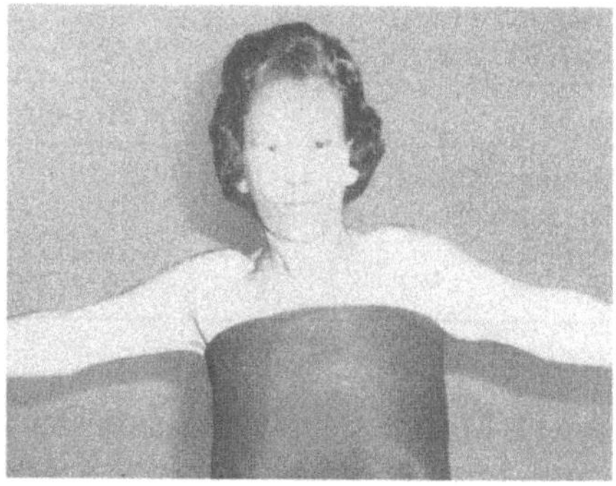

**Fig. 9.** Abduction after removal of right total shoulder replacement

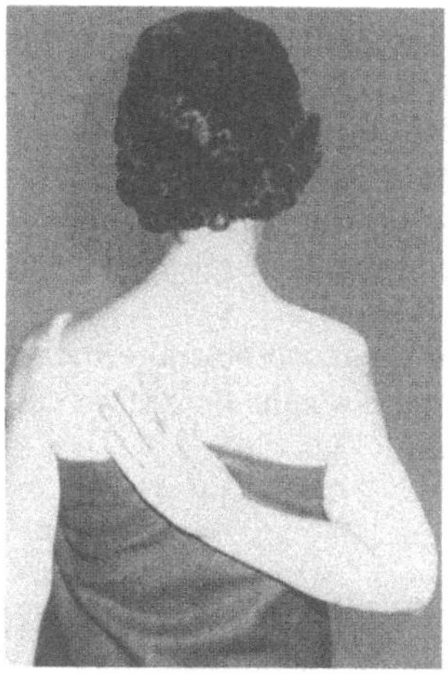

**Fig. 10.** Internal rotation after removal of loose right total shoulder replacement

tion of the average preoperative range of movement in the Neer series, which adds to the difficulties of comparing results (Table 4).

The exclusion of the most seriously affected patients clearly biases the results. It is essential when comparing the results of any form of treatment to compare like with like, and the patients should come from the same statistical population.

Nevertheless, none of the prostheses in Neer's series have come loose (although 30% have developed radiolucent lines around the glenoid component), and 2 years ago we decided to use this prosthesis in our rheumatoid patients with severe pain and gross limitation of glenohumeral movement, for whom we previously would have used the Stanmore shoulder.

The small series of 20 patients reported by Fisher in 1983 suggests that the improvement in range of motion with the Neer prosthesis in rheumatoid patients with severely limited preoperative movement is similar to that achieved by replacement with the Stanmore prosthesis.

My own limited experience with the Neer prosthesis in the last two years confirms this observation. So far only one patient has gained an almost full range of pain-free elevation with the Neer replacement, but internal rotation remains very

**Table 4.** Average Gain in Range of Movement with the Neer Prosthesis. IR Internal Rotation, ER External Rotation

| | | Flexion | Extension | Abduction | IR | ER |
|---|---|---|---|---|---|---|
| Rheum. arthritis | 33% | 57° | ? | ? | ? | 60° |
| Osteoarthritis | 30% | 77° | ? | ? | ? | 51° |
| Post-trauma | 26% | 33° | ? | ? | ? | 58° |
| Revision | 11% | 39° | ? | ? | ? | 51° |

limited. Most patients are able to elevate the arm only to shoulder level, and rarely above. Internal rotation remains limited, but external rotation improves.

Fifty-seven percent of the replacements reported by Neer and his colleagues were performed for primary and secondary osteoarthritis, and I believe this accounts for much of the discrepancy in the range of movement. In Great Britain, shoulder replacement is usually reserved for seriously disabled patients suffering from polyarticular disease. The rotator cuff is usually destroyed in these patients, and its stabilizing action seems to be crucial in restoring movement above shoulder level.

Arthrodesis is preferred for most patients with posttraumatic arthritis, but we have occasionally used the Stanmore prosthesis with satisfactory results.

To date we have not had to revise a Neer prosthesis, but our numbers are still small and our follow-up less than two years. We will continue to use it until we at least have sufficient numbers to compare with our previous series.

The absence of loosening clearly makes this prosthesis an acceptable alternative to arthrodesis in the short term, but we must await long-term results before we can recommend the general use of total shoulder replacement.

## References

1. Fisher WD (1983) The Neer II glenohumeral replacement in the arthritic shoulder. Abstracts from Xth European Congress of Rheumatology, June 26-July 2, Moscow, 250
2. Lettin AWF, Copeland SA, Scales JT (1982) The Stanmore total shoulder replacement. J Bone Joint Surg [Br] 64: 47-51
3. Neer CS (1974) Replacement arthroplasty for glenohumeral osteoarthritis. J Bone Joint Surg [Am] 56: 1-13
4. Neer CS, Watson KC, Stanton FJ (1982) Recent experience in total shoulder replacement. J Bone Joint Surg [Am] 64: 319-336

## Discussion

*Chairman:* The Stanmore prosthesis was the first total shoulder implant, and experience gained with it has benefitted the prostheses of the second generation. But we should not place too much importance on the type of the prosthesis itself. A great deal depends on operative technique and postoperative care.

Dr. Watson, can you say something more about the range of rotational movement before and after operation?

*Watson:* Internal rotation is very important. It is achieved more easily in many of our patients because it plays such a major role in the activities of daily life. External rotation is neccessary for overhead work. Without adequate external rotation, it is extremely difficult to raise the arm above shoulder level. We place great value on internal rotation and find it easier to achieve than external rotation. We cannot expect patients with rheumatoid arthritis and severe rotator deficits to have results as good as other patients. We place our rheumatoid patients and others on an abducting and elevating splint for 3-6 weeks postoperatively, and we have found on mobilizing from the splint that rheumatoid shoulders have a much greater tendency to become stiff than the shoulders of osteoarthritics or patients with posttraumatic conditions.

*Chairman:* What are your views on this, Dr. Lettin?

*Lettin:* We do not place any of our patients on a splint, and we immobilize them for only a minimal period. We try to mobilize our patients as early as possible according to tolerance and with due regard for wound healing. So I cannot say whether the results with another method would be better.

So far I have implanted only 12 Neer prostheses. I started this just under two years ago, and to date we have not been able to restore internal rotation as well as we could with our earlier prosthesis. But perhaps we need to devote a greater amount of effort to rehabilitation.

*Chairman:* We can reconcile this response with Dr. Watson's report by noting that all of Dr. Lettin's comments pertain to patients whom Neer classifies as a "limited goals" group. So everything that Dr. Lettin said is true for that population. All patients who achieved better function belonged to the group which Neer strives to rehabilitate to normal function. This would not be a realistic goal in the rheumatoids of Dr. Lettin's series, who came to operation very late.

Perhaps Prof. Tillmann can shed some light on the question of patient selection.

*Tillmann:* I believe that that the situation in our European centers, which are oriented more toward rheumatoid-orthopedic cases, is different from that at shoulder centers in the United States. We probably operate too late according to U.S. standards. The reason for this is that we see patients who are so multiply disabled that many other indications take precedence over the shoulder, which is at the bottom of the list for reconstructive consideration. This certainly explains why we have more problems with the rotator cuff than our colleagues in the U.S., and correspondingly poorer results. That is why I have developed a new technique of resection arthroplasty, because it creates space and enables me to reconstruct the rotator cuff more effectively. Otherwise I, too, probably would have stayed with prosthetic devices.

*Zippel:* Rotator cuff problems were the impetus for designing a constrained prostheses. In theory this device should eliminate the need for rotator cuff repair, which can be very tedious and may give poor functional results. It yielded the best results when the entire rotator cuff was removed. Unfortunately we have found that, at least with my prosthesis, impingement is a serious problem and can cause the device to break. That has been the problem of the fixed shoulder prosthesis.

*Watson:* Dr. Lettin, can you tell us the percentage of patients with rheumatoid arthritis in whom the rotator cuff was destroyed or completely absent? We have found that soft-tissue restoration is essential to later joint function, but that in many cases the cuff is completely destroyed or irreparable.

*Lettin:* Yes, that is true, and unfortunately we did not document this adequately in the beginning. Since we have done this, however, we have seen extensive and irreversible destruction of the rotator cuff in 60% of cases.

I would like to repeat that my experience with shoulder replacements in nonrheumatoid patients is very limited. In young patients with posttraumatic osteoarthritis affecting only one shoulder, we would prefer to do an arthrodesis. We very rarely see primary osteoarthritis of the shoulder.

The only other comment I can make on this point is that we rarely achieve elevation past 90° despite good rotational movement.

I should emphasize that few activities of daily life involve overhead work. Most tasks are done without raising the arm to 90°. In the early 1970s our first 13 patients were carefully tested by our occupational therapist to assess their function. External rotation is very rarely needed for the activities of daily living, and almost all ordinary tasks are performed in front of the body, below shoulder level, except for putting on clothes and washing the back.

Although we do not obtain significant gains of motion with the Stanmore and Neer prosthesis, we feel that the operation is still justified because of the pain relief that is obtained, which itself improves joint function.

*Pahle:* Dr. Lettin, one question concerning the strategy of operative treatment and the decision whether to perform a Neer arthroplasty or an arthrodesis: Did I understand you to say that you first try to close the rotator cuff rupture, and that if this is not possible you dispense with arthroplasty and perform an arthrodesis?

*Lettin:* No, you did not understand me correctly. I consider arthrodesis inappropriate in rheumatoids, because multiple joints are affected by the disease. The joint involvement in rheumatoid arthritis is usually symmetrical. When one shoulder is involved, the other one usually is, too. Therefore I would not advocate arthrodesis of the shoulder for rheumatoid patients, and I always replace the joint regardless of whether I can rebuild the rotator cuff. We use arthrodesis for monoarticular problems, which are usually posttraumatic at our center.

*Chairman:* Concerning the range of postoperative rotation: Have you found that the limitation of external rotation relates to the design of the Stanmore prosthesis or to the reattachment of the subscapularis?

*Lettin:* Initially we reefed the subscapularis on the assumption that dislocation would be a problem. Thus we intentionally limited external rotation in our early patients. But when we had no problems with dislocation, we discontinued that practice. I do not believe that limitation of external rotation was due to impingement of the prosthesis, but rather to contracture and scarring of the soft tissues. We used an image intensifier to investigate this in our patients.

We all know that shoulders become stiff very rapidly after surgery or trauma. The stiffness appears to be a natural circumstance, and we may be too optimistic if we think that we can always achieve a complete range of motion.

# Shoulder Replacement Arthroplasty

J. A. Pahle*

Synovectomy of the shoulder joint has been performed at the Oslo Sanitetsforening Rheumatism Hospital since 1968 and has given satisfactory results even in advanced cases [5, 8]. In a recent review of 54 shoulder synovectomies with an average follow-up of 5.3 years (1-16 years), synovectomy was found to provide lasting benefit even in advanced cases. Twenty-six of these cases were classified as grade III according to the system of Larsen et al. (1977) and required debridement in addition to synovectomy [9]. Only six of these shoulders later required total prosthetic replacement.

Arthrodesis may give good results [11] when scapulothoracic motion is well preserved, but in our experience this is seldom the case in rheumatoid arthritis. The relatively small contact surfaces left in cases of severe destruction will jeopardize solid bony healing, and the osteogenic potential in rheumatoid arthritis may be greatly diminished. This means that bone healing will require lengthy immobilization, which poses a danger to affected neighboring joints. We consider arthrodesis of the shoulder joint to be necessary in cases where heavy weight bearing on the shoulder is anticipated, as in patients who have to rely permanently on crutches. This aspect may strengthen the indications for reconstructive operations on the lower extremities.

The results after insertion of a total prosthesis are encouraging [2], and arthrodesis has not proved necessary at our hospital since 1973.

## Material and Methods

Between 1973 and 1984 we replaced 64 shoulders in 56 patients at our center. The patients consisted of 45 women and 11 men ranging in age from 22 to 72 years (average 50.3 years). Three patients suffered from ankylosing spondylitis and two from juvenile rheumatoid arthritis. The remaining 51 all had rheumatoid arthritis. The mean duration of disease was 18.7 years and thus considerably longer than in synovectomy cases, where the average disease duration was 10.5 years. One of the shoulders represents the reversal of an arthrodesis into a reasonably well functioning joint. Most of the cases were in radiologically advanced stages (Fig. 1):

| | | |
|---|---|---|
| Preoperative radiographic findings: | Grade III | 2 |
| (after Larsen et al. [3a]) | Grade IV | 31 |
| | Grade V | 31. |

Only five of these shoulders had undergone previous synovectomy. Thirty-five of the patients were being treated with corticosteroids. Eight patients had both shoulder joints replaced.

---

* This paper is based on an article appearing in *Ann Chir Gynaecol 74*/198 (1985) [9]. This revised version is published with the permission of the special editor.

Shoulder Replacement
Eds.: Kölbel/Helbig/Blauth

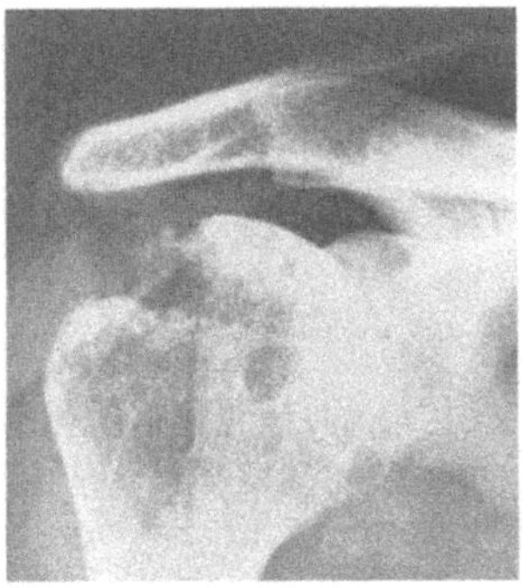

**Fig. 1.** Advanced case of rheumatoid arthritis, with cysts on the verge of penetration

The semiconstrained prosthesis of Lettin-Stanmore [4] was used in the first 13 patients. Fixation of the glenoid component of the Lettin prosthesis is technically difficult in rheumatoid patients, whose bone stock may be greatly reduced. We abandoned this model when the unconstrained Engelbrecht-St. Georg prosthesis was introduced in 1978. Engelbrecht's radical approach to the joint, involving division of the subscapularis, supraspinatus, infraspinatus, and teres minor tendons, made insertion of the prosthetic components easy, but we found it quite difficult to close the rotator cuff and reattach it to the brittle osteoporotic bone in rheumatoid patients. We used the Engelbrecht-St. Georg prosthesis in 10 cases. In advanced rheumatoid cases, upward migration of the head of the humerus, very often combined with "medialization," will limit the number of cases suitable for this type of prosthesis due to the rather large head size of the humeral component. The constriction of the rotator cuff in these cases simply does not leave the space necessary for the prosthesis (Fig. 2). This prosthesis comes in only one size.

There is clearly a need for several stem sizes, and a smaller size prosthesis is needed in patients suffering from *juvenile* chronic arthritis.

The two head sizes and six stem sizes available in the Neer II prosthesis [7] were decisive in 1979 when we felt it necessary to change to a new prosthesis:

| | |
|---|---|
| 1973-1977 Lettin-Stanmore | 13 |
| 1978-1979 Engelbrecht-St. Georg | 10 |
| 1979-1984 Neer II | 41 |

## Surgical Technique

The surgeon undertaking a shoulder replacement arthroplasty should be well versed in general surgery of the shoulder and especially in soft-tissue repair [7]. More often than not, the rotator cuff is damaged by the disease.

The patient is placed in the supine position with the shoulder elevated on a firm cushion and the arm abducted on a side table. Neer's long deltopectoral approach is recommended for arthroplasty as well as for synovectomy of the shoulder. Sometimes the clavicular part of the deltoid must be released from its origin, but usually the anterior part of the deltoid can be retracted far enough superiorly and posteriorly with Hohmann retractors to expose the rotator cuff and proximal humerus without this additional release. It is wise to divide the cranial part of the pectoralis major tendon, and division of the coracoacromial ligament is sometimes necessary. The

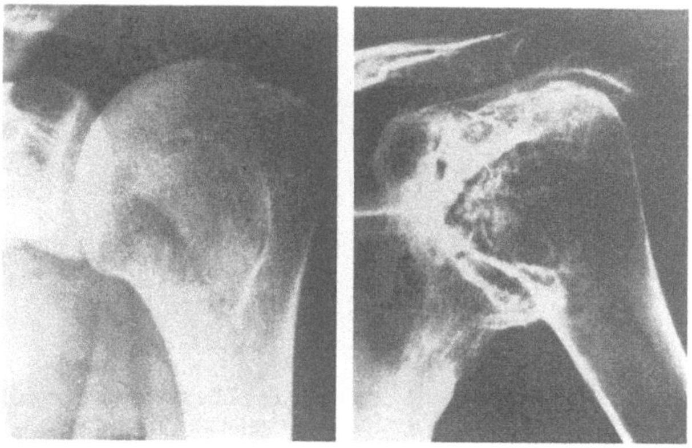

**Fig. 2.** Superomedial displacement of the head

subacromial and subdeltoid bursae may now be excised if they are found to be inflamed. Synovectomy of the acromioclavicular joint is performed if required. The tendon of the long head of the biceps is inspected in its bicipital groove, and tenosynovectomy is performed [8]. In most cases this tendon has been found ruptured, usually with its distal stump adherent to periosteum in the bicipital groove. If this is not the case, the distal stump should be sutured to the transverse ligament. The proximal stump may be used to repair defects of the rotator cuff.

Meticulous preparation of the subscapularis tendon should be done before the tendon is divided, the medial stump being secured with holding sutures. This preparation should include freeing of muscular adhesions to the anterior glenoid margin to ensure a freely functioning subscapularis muscle after reattachment. A pull on the proximal stump should elicit a springy resistance as a sign of muscle tonus.

After the joint is opened, retractors are introduced intraarticularly. The joint surfaces are usually well visualized once adhesions are cleared, and a final decision can be made between synovectomy and prosthetic replacement. If the surfaces are still spherical and the subchondral cortical bone smooth, a synovectomy with debridement may give good lasting results even if the cartilage is entirely absent. The head resection should be made as sparingly as possible, and the osteotomy plane should be oriented in 40° of retroversion, using a trial prosthesis as a guide. In juvenile rheumatoid arthritis, however, the growth disturbances that are so prevalent in this disease may have resulted in loss of anteversion of the glenoid joint surface, sometimes even to the 0° position, and the osteotomy plane of the humerus will have to be changed correspondingly.

The frequent upward migration seen in rheumatoid patients makes it difficult to obtain good centering of the prosthetic components unless a larger portion of the humeral head is resected. In the last two years we have developed a modification of the Neer II prosthesis in which the lateral perforated fin has been removed, and the remaining three fins have been reduced in width to fit in the narrower distal part of the neck of the humerus, thus avoiding fractures in the osteoporotic bone.

In adults, where osteoporosis is pronounced, the medullary canal is usually wide. In juvenile rheumatoids, on the other hand, the diaphysis is slender and can accommodate only the 6.3-mm stem. The glenoid may be exposed by means of a Bankart retractor held carefully to avoid damaging the brittle bone. In this way the posterior part of the neck of the glenoid can be defined. Granulation tissue and remnants of

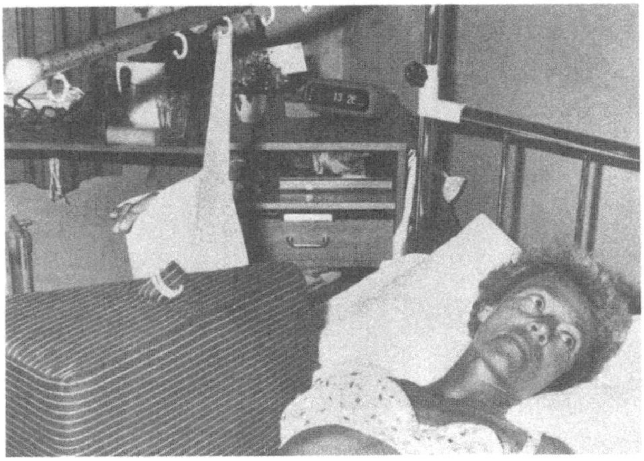

**Fig. 3.** The arm is suspended in a "gallows." The abduction pillow is used when the patient is ambulatory

labrum are removed to visualize the whole circumference of the articular surface, which should be carefully trimmed to ensure a snug fit of the glenoid prosthesis. The slot for the stem of the glenoid component is cut with a ball reamer, and the edge is undercut with small curettes. A concentric row of drill holes is made in the cortex of the articular surface to improve cement dispersion. We have used the standard polyethylene glenoid component *without* a metal backing in all of our patients, for we feel that the polyethylene gives a more natural transition to the "soft" rheumatic bone. Great care should be taken to ensure a stable fit of the glenoid component even before it is cemented into place. Preferably the two components should be tested together several times to ensure good centering and stable position.

The definitive glenoid component is cemented first. The humeral component should be tested again in situ before it is cemented. Tears of the rotator cuff are repaired, possibly using portions of the supraspinatus tendon and the proximal stump of the long head of the biceps. The subscapularis tendon is sutured to the lateral stump or to drill holes in the cortex (and through the cement if necessary). Approximating sutures are placed in the deltoid and pectoralis major muscles; suction drainage is maintained for 24h.

With this *minimal* muscle release advocated by Neer, in which usually only the subscapularis tendon is divided, postoperative immobilization has been shortened to a couple of days with the arm suspended in a "gallows" (Fig. 3). Afterward active isometric exercises are instituted with the arm resting on an abduction pillow. Assisted dynamic exercises are usually started after 10-14 days. The training is aimed at obtaining a good muscular balance to secure centering of the ball and socket prosthesis.

## Results

The need for 3 weeks' immobilization in a Velpeau bandage following Lettin's approach made postoperative training difficult, especially with regard to abduction. After introduction of the Engelbrecht prosthesis, the arm was immobilized on an abduction splint for three weeks. During this time isometric exercises of the external

**Table 1.** Postoperative Gain of Motion in 64 Shoulders, in Degrees

| | Lettin-Stanmore | St. Georg-Engelbrecht | Neer |
|---|---|---|---|
| Abduction | 9.6 | 13.9 | 24 |
| Flexion | −4.2 | 7.8 | 16 |
| Extension | 3.5 | 14.4 | 12.9 |
| External rotation | 1.2 | 13.9 | 14.6 |
| Internal rotation | 5.4 | 22.2 | 6.5 |
| Length of follow-up (years) | 9 | 5.6 | 3.2 |

**Table 2.** Complications

| | Lettin-Stanmore (n=13) | St. Georg-Engelbrecht (n=10) | Neer (n=41) |
|---|---|---|---|
| Primary infection | 0 | 0 | 1 |
| Loosening and late infection | 2 | 0 | 1 |
| Loosening without infection | 3 | 2 | 1 |
| Fracture of humerus | 2 | 0 | 1 |
| Fracture of glenoid | 1 | 0 | 0 |
| Dislocation | 0 | 0 | 1 |
| Technical failure | 0 | 0 | 5 |

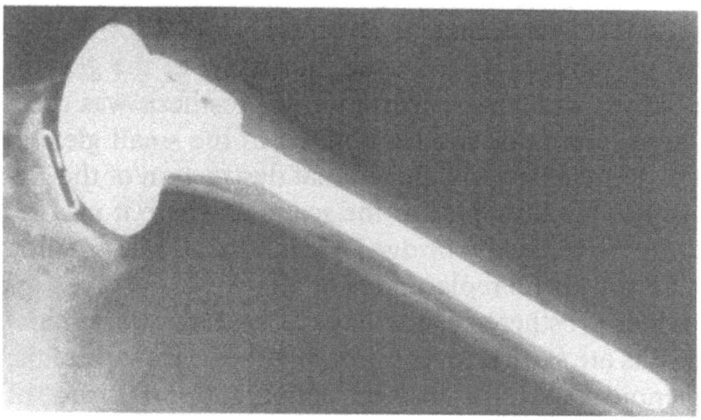

**Fig. 4.** Satisfactory centering of the head

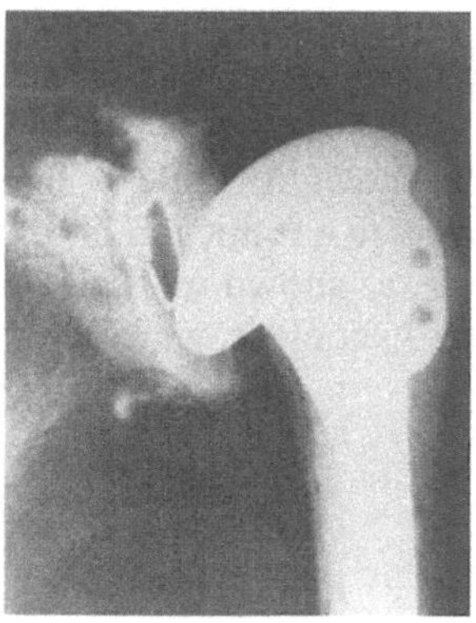

**Fig. 5.** Superior migration of the head

**Table 3.** Assessment of Results by the Patients

| | Better | Same | Worse |
|---|---|---|---|
| Pain | 51 | 7 | 6 |
| Range of motion | 44 | 14 | 6 |
| Function | 48 | 11 | 5 |

**Table 4.** Perception of Pain before and after Operation

| | Lettin-Stanmore (n=13) | St. Georg-Engelbrecht (n=10) | Neer (n=41) |
|---|---|---|---|
| Preoperative pain | 13 | 9 | 41 |
| Postoperative pain | 5 | 2 | 6 |

and internal rotators and the deltoid were performed twice daily. Thereafter the range of motion increased rapidly.

As Table 1 shows, a gain in motion was obtained in all cases except for the 13 patients who had been treated with the Lettin-Stanmore prosthesis; most of the latter patients displayed a a moderate loss of flexion postoperatively. The range of motion is the active motion, while abduction denotes the total range of abduction of the upper extremity. No separate measurement was made of the glenohumeral contribution to abduction. It matters little to the patient whether or not this abduction occurs as a combined movement; it is the total range that counts.

The complications are listed in Table 2. As expected, loosening of the glenoid component occurred most frequently when a semiconstrained prosthesis was used. This is due to the relatively large forces that are transmitted to the small glenoid component from the upper arm. It must be remembered that destruction of the glenoid cavity sometimes extends into the thin neck of the scapula, where it may reduce the bony cover of the socket to a narrow bridge [10]. In fact, the destruction may be too advanced to permit a prosthetic replacement at all.

Our experience with 41 shoulder prostheses of the Neer II type can be summarized as follows: The overall results are satisfactory (Fig. 4), but the oval shape of the head together with the small glenoid socket that lacks the cranial support (fornix) of the Engelbrecht-St. Georg design, mimicking normal anatomy, makes it difficult to center the components properly. Tissue contraction in the postoperative course can lead to upward migration of the head (Fig. 5), giving a result that was classified as a technical failure in 5 cases (see Table 2).

The subjective assessment of the results by the patients is shown in Table 3. The best results in terms of pain relief, which in most cases permitted a reduction of analgesic medication, were obtained with the Neer prosthesis, as shown in Table 4. Twelve patients stated that they could not lie on the operated shoulder, which they perceived as a significant limitation.

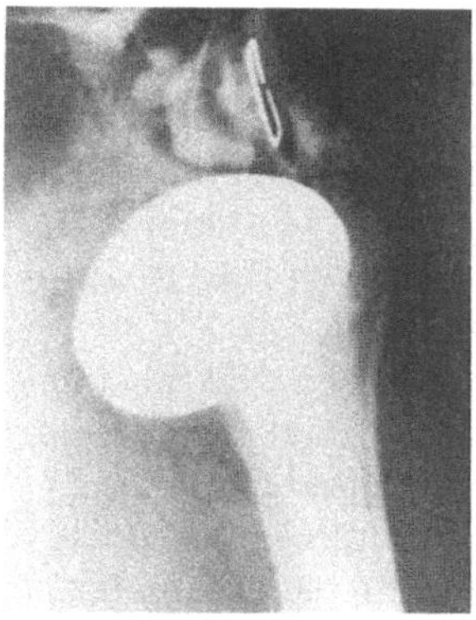

**Fig. 6.** Distal dislocation following rupture of the supraspinatus muscle

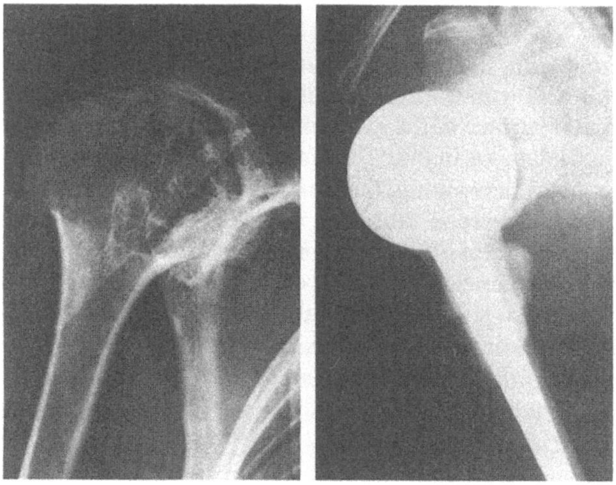

**Fig. 7.** In juvenile rheumatoid arthritis, special stem designs may be required for the narrow humeral shaft

## Discussion

The main problems in shoulder replacement arthroplasty for *rheumatoid arthritis* relate to the ever-present osteoporosis caused by the disease itself (vasculitis?), the widespread use of corticosteroids, and inactivity. The small and often severely damaged articular surface of the glenoid aggravates the problem of fixation. Even if the unconstrained prosthesis is theoretically preferable in the shoulder as it is in other joints, destruction of the rotator cuff with loss of its stabilizing function sometimes makes it necessary to use a semiconstrained device that possesses some amount of intrinsic stability [4, 10].

It should be remembered, however, that the transmission of forces from one part of the prosthesis to the other is unavoidable. The latest generation of prostheses work on the principle of the unconstrained replacement, which often demands a technically difficult functional restoration of the rotator cuff and deltoid. Only when there is ideal coordination of the deltoid and rotator cuff muscles will the resultant force pass through the center of the joint in all positions of the humerus. Normally the distance between the acromion and the humerus is exactly what is necessary for the greater tuberosity to pass beneath the acromion during abduction [1]. If the rotator cuff is destroyed, the head will move superiorly, and abduction will be blocked. Without a functioning supraspinatus muscle, the humeral head will tend to dislocate inferiorly when a weight is exerted on the dependent arm (Fig. 6).

A prosthesis cannot function without a "motor." The necessity of a well-functioning rotator cuff and deltoid [6] implies that an unconstrained total replacement should *not* be tried as a late salvage operation after other procedures have failed.

The ideal shoulder prosthesis should restore sufficient motion for normal daily activities, especially in rotation [3]. It is seldom necessary for the patient to abduct the shoulder more than 90° if the elbow joint is functioning well. *Internal* rotation is of much greater importance. The range of motion is determined mainly by the position of the two halves of the prosthesis, which in turn depends strongly on the remaining bone stock.

As Kölbel et al. [3] have pointed out, the *center of motion* of the natural shoulder joint is located about 10 mm medial to the longitudinal axis of the humerus and about 25 mm lateral to the articular surface of the glenoid. Thus, the ideal prosthesis should offer an assortment of neck lengths in both the humeral and glenoid components, and at least two different head sizes should be available. Multiple stem thicknesses are necessary to avoid thermal necrosis caused by a thick layer of cement in a wide medullary canal. Cementless fixation of the components in advanced cases of rheumatoid arthritis may give uncertain results due to compromise of osteogenic potential. A great need exists for a design that can meet the specific demands of the dysplastic humeral heads and shafts in *juvenile* rheumatoid arthritis (Fig. 7). The ideal prosthesis should be unconstrained, but at the same time it should provide a cranial support that can check the tendency of upward migration of the head and maintain concentricity of the joint.

With improvements in technique, the "technical failures" in our material probably can be avoided. Eight of the operations were bilateral, reflecting the patients' satisfaction with the procedure. The greatest benefits from the patients' standpoint are pain relief, the ability to sleep on the operated shoulder, increased internal rotation allowing perineal hygiene, flexion enabling hair grooming, and adduction enabling the patient to reach the contralateral axillary fossa.

## References

1. Crossan JF, Vallance R (1982) The shoulder joint in rheumatoid arthritis. Manuscript 1982.
2. Kessel L, Bayley I (1979) Prosthetic replacement of shoulder joint: Preliminary communication. J R Soc Med 72: 748-752
3. Kölbel R, Rohlmann A, Bergmann G, Friedebold G (1977) Shoulder joint replacement: Kölbel-Friedebold-method. In: Burri C, Coldewey J, Rüter A (eds) Endoprostheses and alternatives for the arm. Shoulder joint. Huber, Bern pp 47-60

3a. Larsen A, Dale K, Eek M (1977) Radiographic evaluation of rheumatoid arthritis and related conditions by standard reference films. Acta Radiol [Diagn] (Stockh) 18: 481-491

4. Lettin A (1981) Shoulder replacement in rheumatoid arthritis. In: Goldie IF (ed) Surgery in rheumatoid arthritis, reconstruction surgery and traumatology, vol 18. Karger, Basel, pp 55-62

5. Neer CS (1971) The rheumatoid shoulder, surgery of rheumatoid arthritis. Lippincott, Philadelphia, pp 117-125
6. gestrichen
7. Neer CS, Watson KE, Stanton FJ (1982) Recent experience in total shoulder replacement. J Bone Joint Surg [Am] 64 3: 319-337
8. Pahle JA (1981) The shoulder joint in rheumatoid arthritis: Synovectomy. In: Goldie IF (ed) Surgery in rheumatoid arthritis, reconstruction surgery and traumatology, vol 18. Karger, Basel, pp 33-47
9. Pahle JA, Kvarnes L (1985) Shoulder synovectomy. Ann Chir Gynaecol [Suppl] 74/198: 37-39
10. Post M, Jablon M, Miller H, Singh M (1979) Constrained total shoulder joint replacement: A critical review. Clin Orthop 144: 135-150
11. Raunio P (1981) Arthrodesis of the shoulder joint in rheumatoid arthritis. In: Goldie IF (ed) Surgery in rheumatoid arthritis, reconstruction surgery and traumatology, vol 18. Karger, Basel, pp 48-54

## Discussion

*Blauth:* You referred to five cases of technical failure in connection with superior migration of the head of the humerus or prosthesis. What were the errors leading to the failures?

*Pahle:* One involved faulty positioning or tilting of the glenoid component; another apparently involved failure to resect the proximal humerus at the correct level. I simply do not believe that it is sufficient to resect a small cap from the humeral head. In most cases of rheumatoid arthritis the disease has caused superior displacement of the humeral head, and this makes it necessary to resect more bone. (Editor's note: With reference to the reports of Welsh and Cofield, it is noted that relative positioning of the humerus and glenoid is achieved by releasing the capsule. Afterward one needs to resect only as much of the deformed upper humerus as is necessary to insert the prosthesis and correctly position the head.)

Superior displacement of the head prosthesis was due mainly to the fact that we did not seat the glenoid component at the proper inclination.

*N. N.:* Can you tell us more about when you would perform a late synovectomy, and when you would insert a prosthesis?

*Pahle:* I believe that a final decision cannot be made until the joint has been opened. The patient should understand this and should give the surgeon his consent for making this decision. The findings at operation may be worse than the X-rays indicated, or they may be better. If the joint surfaces are smooth and the head and glenoid are reasonably spherical, I would not insert a total prosthesis even if all the cartilage were gone. The long-term results of synovectomy in these advanced cases are very convincing, in the shoulder as well as in the knee. At present we are concluding a study of 10-year results in these patients. You know what happens to total knee replacements after a few years: They tend to become loose.

*Chairman:* Yesterday I presented a case of disseminated lupus erythematosus and said that I considered the risk of infection in such patients, who may be taking cytostatics and cortisone, to be prohibitive for joint replacement. What is your position?

*Pahle:* My view is that many of these patients have a short life expectancy, and that that should not discourage us from giving them the best treatment possible. It is not the length of life that counts, but its quality. The woman I described had absolutely no use of her arm, and we wanted to improve that situation. We told her that the risks were very high, as we have in other cases in which a very good result was obtained later. In this case we did not expect that the prosthesis would fail so quickly, but it is good to be reminded that one should consider all the possible consequences before inserting a total prosthesis.

# Comments on Joint Replacement in Rheumatoid Arthritis

R. H. Cofield

Rheumatoid arthritis of the shoulder presents as a spectrum of pathology. Primary involvement seems to be of the synovial and bursal tissues. Secondary involvement includes many tissues, most notably the cartilage, tendons, and bone. Laine et al. [2] reviewed the shoulder affections in rheumatoid arthritis and found a variety of soft tissues and joints involved. Our patients have presented with extreme bursal disease only, intensive synovitis with very few other changes, predominant rotator cuff disease, predominant cartilage loss, or a combination of these lesions.

In reviewing our patients with rheumatoid shoulder disease requiring surgery, we found that many different procedures were employed, but that the great majority involved some form of prosthetic replacement. As shoulder replacement arthroplasty became more widely practiced, its application to rheumatoid disease in the shoulder became a much more significant part of the care of the rheumatoid patient. Our typical patient presented with cartilage loss associated with pain and limited function and then underwent a total shoulder arthroplasty. We performed many associated procedures in this group of patients, including synovectomy, acromioplasty, rotator cuff repair, bursectomy, and excision of the distal clavicle. In our patients who required replacement arthroplasty between 1976 and 1981, 29.7% had some degree of rotator cuff tearing. This figure is considerably below that reported by Rybka [3] in patients undergoing arthrodesis but is consistent with that reported by Ennevarra [1] in an arthrographic study of rheumatoid shoulders. If a rotator cuff tear exists, the most common means of closing it when repair is done in conjunction with arthroplasty is the procedure of subscapularis transposition.

Arthrodesis has been proposed as an alternative to total shoulder arthroplasty for these patients. We often consider this procedure, but we almost never do it. The functional capabilities of a patient with an arthrodesis are much below those of a patient with a total shoulder replacement, and the need for revision surgery in rheumatoid patients with total shoulder implants is quite low. This may well relate to the low stresses placed upon the implant.

Polyarticular involvement is very common in rheumatoid patients. Surgical sequencing has been a philosophical item for discussion. Of course if there is neurologic change, especially when significant or progressive, cervical stabilization is considered before other procedures. We generally reconstruct the lower extremity first if there is substantial disability before turning our attention to the upper extremity. It is possible to do a shoulder procedure and a minor hand procedure at the same operation, but I feel it is too much to combine a shoulder procedure with an elbow procedure or with a major hand procedure at one sitting. We now believe that it makes no difference whether the shoulder or the elbow is done first when both joints require surgical care. If the elbow is done first, often the cement extends quite far proximally into the humerus. One must be aware of this so that the humeral prosthesis can be suitably shortened at the time of surgery.

There are three situations in which prosthetic humeral head replacement should

Shoulder Replacement
Eds.: Kölbel/Helbig/Blauth

be considered in preference to total shoulder replacement in patients with rheumatoid arthritis:

1) significant medial resorption of the scapula,
2) extreme osteoporosis,
3) oligoarticular disease in a younger patient.

We are now quite cautious about performing a hemiarthroplasty in a young patient with oligoarticular disease, for we have been unable to predict who will and who will not achieve adequate pain relief.

The last point I wish to make about rheumatoid arthritis of the shoulder is that the extent of pathologic changes varies over time. If the symptoms suggest that shoulder replacement may be beneficial but are not severe enough to make the procedure mandatory, one might wish to inform the patient that further destruction might occur, and that this will make later surgery much more difficult and will compromise the end result.

In summary, many tissue changes occur in the rheumatoid shoulder that have relevance to its surgical management. The synovium may become hypertrophic and scarred, and it may require release at the time of surgery. The bone becomes osteoporotic and often resorbs. Of particular importance to shoulder replacement is the resorption that occurs in the scapula. The tendons are also involved. Tendon tearing occurs in one-fourth to one-third of patients who require prosthetic replacement, but attrition of the tendons with thinning and stretching is a more common feature of glenohumeral disease and may affect the final outcome as far as movement and strength are concerned. Many surgical options exist, but we have found that a prosthesis is usually necessary in patients who require operation. Hemiarthroplasty is an option in some situations, but total shoulder replacement is most useful for the majority of patients, as it provides excellent pain relief, facilitates rehabilitation, and affords a greater gain of motion. Also, it appears that the stresses placed on the implant are low in these patients, and that the loosening rate is also quite low.

## References


1. Ennevarra K (1967) Painful shoulder joint in rheumatoid arthritis. Acta Rheumatol Scand [Suppl] 11
2. Laine VAI, Vainio KJ, Pekanmaki K (1954) Shoulder affections in rheumatoid arthritis. Ann Rheum Dis 13: 157-160
3. Rybka V, Raunio P, Vainio K (1979) Arthrodesis of the shoulder in rheumatoid arthritis. J Bone Joint Surg [Br] 61: 155-158

## Discussion

*Blauth:* We have seen that the crux of the problem is the rotator cuff, and I would like to ask Dr. Cofield if he has any special tricks or suggestions, such as releasing the supraspinatus from the supraspinous fossa.

*Cofield:* In rheumatoids as in other patients with cuff tears, it is important to ascertain what is reactive scar tissue and what is tendon. This is difficult in rheumatoid arthritis, because the tendons themselves are often scarred and present more the appearance of scar tissue than the ordered fibrous structure of tendons. Once the surgeon has distinguished scar tissue from tendon, he should deal with the rotator cuff as he would in any other patient. In about two-thirds of patients with cuff tears, the tears are more or less longitudinal. This is not a serious problem and can be managed by suturing tendon to tendon. But if the tendons are torn in the other direction, one must attach the tendon to the bone over a prosthesis, which then must have a smaller head. If the defect is large, there are established methods of closing it such as McLaughlin's V-Y plasty with attachment to the humeral head. This is not possible, of course, when a prosthesis has been inserted, and one of the other two methods must be chosen. Concerning the transposition of an entire muscle, such as releasing the supraspinatus and transferring it laterally as one would transfer a free flap on a vascular pedicle, this is probably not necessary. One can release the upper and lower surface of the muscle through the tear with a periosteal elevator and then transpose the muscle without exposing it completely. Probably the most practical solution is to transpose the tendinous insertions. This can be done with the subscapularis by mobilzing it at its inferior surface and borders and then pulling it upward. The same applies to the infraspinatus, which comes from the opposite direction and which can be mobilized downward to the axillary nerve. Another method is to patch the cuff tear with a free graft, but I no longer do this. I no longer consider it a good method and would recommend the tendon transfer.

# Shoulder Replacement in Posttraumatic Conditions, Osteoarthritis, and Arthropathies

# Indications and Considerations of Shoulder Replacement in Posttraumatic Conditions

K.C. Watson

Posttraumatic degeneration of the shoulder is one of the more difficult categories with which to deal when considering replacement surgery. On the whole, these patients tend to be young, they are disabled at an active and productive time in their lives, and the demands and stresses they will subsequently place on the prosthesis will be greater and of longer duration than those anticipated for the older osteoarthritic and the less active rheumatoid groups. The dominant arm will be involved more frequently, and there will usually have been previous surgery. In addition, these patients are more likely to have partial or complete nerve palsy (especially axillary) as well as bone loss or deformity (e.g., malunion or nonunion). The presence of these complicating factors requires a thorough preoperative assessment including multiple radiographic views or techniques and often electromyographic evaluation. Postinjury pain and scar may mask a partial axillary nerve palsy picked up on electromyography, which could alter the prognosis or the timing of any reconstructive surgery.

In many cases special techniques have to be employed to deal with these problems. Malunion of the tuberosities often requires osteotomy and reorientation of the tuberosities, and uneven wear of the glenoid can require bone grafting or sculpting of the glenoid to achieve an acceptable alignment and seating. Bone deficits in the proximal humerus cannot be tolerated. The expedient of seating the prosthesis on the sturdiest bone available is unacceptable. This would leave the humerus too short, weakening the deltoid and predisposing to instability. Tension must be maintained in the soft-tissue envelope in order to recover deltoid function, and the bone deficit must be reconstructed with grafting.

Contracture and scarring of the rotator cuff is quite common. Use of the short-head prosthesis may be necessary to obtain closure of the rotator cuff and maintain stability. This sacrifices some of the mechanical advantage afforded by the longer head. Internal rotation contracture is also common, and lengthening of the subscapularis by Z-plasty may be necessary to obtain an acceptable passive external rotation.

Muscle deficits of the deltoid most often occur in the anterior part following previous surgery in which a repair of the deltoid origin has pulled loose, or the deltopectoral interval was not found and a portion of the anterior deltoid was denervated. Limited muscle transfers (of the deltoid and pectoralis major) may be useful in obliterating these defects and improving function.

Bracing and special rehabilitative procedures will often be required in these patients. Chronic dislocations, because of their tendency to redislocate after replacement, require more extensive soft-tissue releases, meticulous attention to version (sometimes altering the normal version of the humeral prosthesis), postoperative bracing and protection during the rehabilitation period. Because of the above problems, the posttraumatic patients as a whole have the least improvement in function, and especially in active elevation. However, because of their age and activity level,

Shoulder Replacement
Eds.: Kölbel/Helbig/Blauth

even modest gains in range of motion, when combined with pain relief, can yield a quite acceptable improvement in function.

As with any joint replacement procedure, patient selection is important. There are instances where nerve and bone deficits are so severe that the function obtained with a prosthesis may not be sufficient for the patient's needs, and an alternative treatment such as arthrodesis might be more appropriate.

In summary, there are four special problems to be considered in individuals with posttraumatic arthritis:

1) loss of bone stock,
2) rotator cuff defects,
3) deltoid defects, and
4) chronic dislocations.

Although any of these problems may be encountered in the other diagnostic categories, it is in the posttraumatic group that they tend to predominate and even occur multiply in the same individual. Reconstruction of these shoulders requires special surgical techniques and a superlative experience in shoulder surgery. When performed correctly in the right patients, these procedures can be effective and rewarding.

## References

Neer CS, Watson KC, Stanton FM (1982) Recent experience in total shoulder replacement. J Bone Joint Surg [Am] 64: 319-337

## Discussion

*Chairman:* There are two questions that need to be addressed: whether we should offer joint replacement to patients at the age you mentioned, and whether open reduction and stabilization would have been possible in the patient with a neglected posterior dislocation - especially since the radiograph indicated that the articular surface of the humeral head was still well preserved.

*Watson:* Yes, that would have been appropriate in one case at an earlier stage. One year had elapsed when the patient was referred to us, and the condition of the joint cartilage had deteriorated: It was greatly thinned, and there were areas on the glenoid that were entirely denuded of cartilage. After we had tried to reduce the fracture and the shoulder, which was very difficult, the joint surface of the humeral head was likewise in poor condition. I do not believe that this is the treatment method of choice for recent injuries. The treatment of choice would be to recognize the injury at an earlier stage. Unfortunately, we very often see such injuries when it is already too late.

*Chairman:* There is another problem that I would like to add to the list of cuff tears, deltoid damage, bone loss, etc.: that of posttraumatic adhesions. Based on your experience, is there anything that one must do in order to mobilize the soft tissues?

*Watson:* You should recover as much motion as possible at operation, because there will be no other opportunity where you can accomplish so much. Also, you should start very intensive exercises as early as possible to move the arm passively through the range of motion achieved and thus improve it further. We find continuous passive motion to be very useful. A motorized motion splint, for example, can operate continuously throughout the day, whereas a patient on standard physiotherapy would be exercised only once or twice daily. I do not believe that this significantly improves long-term results, but it makes it easier to recover movement in a short time. For this reason I have not mobilized shoulders under anesthesia after total arthroplasty and in some cases have not achieved a complete range of motion. Postoperative adhesions are more pronounced in patients with old fractures; mobilization is more difficult and requires more time. We are speaking here of 9 months to a year in some cases, and the active and passive ranges may still increase further after that time.

*Marti:* I had the impression in one case that the humeral head prosthesis was loose. It seemed to pump up and down in the bone. If that were the case, how would you handle such a problem? Does it cause pain, or do you disregard it?

*Watson:* The prosthesis did not move up and down in the humerus, but rather with the humerus relative to the scapula. I believe that in the case you refer to, the woman had significant weakness of the deltoid. We had not expected that she would recover her mobility so well. The patient was pain free, and she is very pleased with the result. With greater subluxation, the problem becomes very difficult to manage. There are patients with rotator defects in whom the prosthesis goes on to migrate under the clavicle. We do not really have a good solution for these cases. Removing the prosthesis will not solve the problem, for then the humeral shaft will continue to move in the same manner and direction. Reconstructing the tuberosities with bone grafts and attaching the rotator cuff to them has given only temporary success because of subsequent resorption of the grafts. So this is an area that we are still working on. Unfortunately, as the numbers of shoulder replacements increase, we will have to face this problem even more often in the future.

*Blauth:* Having spoken to us about your indications and the technical aspects of joint replacement for post-trauma cases, could you also tell us how many patients you are following, how long you have followed them, what complications you have seen, and what your results are?

*Watson:* We have followed our patients for quite some time. We first saw them every week, then every two weeks, then once a month, and so on. Thereafter they return each year for a clinical and X-ray examination. The results have been very acceptable as far as pain relief is concerned. As for function, this has been improved. Our X-ray evaluations have not shown significant deterioration. Function has been maintained well, and in fact many patients whom we see at one year and then at two years are doing better after the second year than after the first.

*Chairman:* Prof. Blauth's question pertained to the large series that you published with Dr. Neer in 1982. Would you tell us again how many of these patients were post-trauma cases?

*Watson:* I believe 46 were. About 1/3 to 1/2 of them had really good results. Two-thirds had satisfactory to excellent results, and the remaining 1/3 had less than satisfactory results. I believe that the three patients from the series who reported no subjective improvement were not part of the post-trauma group.

*Blauth:* Have you changed your indications in comparison with 3 or 5 years ago?

*Watson:* As we gain more experience and more confidence in the longevity of the replacement, we become less hesitant about using it in younger patients, especially since they are in an active period of their lives. I cannot contradict your statement that one would do just as well or better with an arthrodesis in monoarticular cases as far as longevity is concerned. The question of whether the dominant or nondominant arm is involved also has to be considered. But in the case of a young person whose dominant arm is affected, causing pain and limiting his ability to work, I would urge prosthetic reconstruction. Conversion to an arthrodesis would be possible if reoperation becomes necessary. It is not simple, but it can give a reasonably good result.

*N. N.:* In the earlier works of Neer, comminuted fractures and fracture-dislocations were recognized as indications for joint replacement arthroplasty. This group seems to be underrepresented in the present series. How specifically do you deal with a comminuted fracture-dislocation in a 50-year-old patient?

*Watson:* With significant tuberosity displacement that disrupts the blood supply to the joint surface, we would do a reconstruction with a prosthesis. If the tuberosities are fractured but not displaced, we could treat the case nonoperatively or by rigid internal fixation. This would not be an indication for a prosthesis. Displacement of the fragments is the key consideration. I believe that the blood supply is adequate, for example, when one tuberosity is markedly displaced but the head is intact and maintains contact with the other tuberosity. In that case the joint surface would still be adequately supplied through the undisplaced tuberosity. This would be an indication for nonprosthetic reconstruction. So, we reserve the prosthesis for very specific types of fracture (Editor's note: 4-part fractures with significant displacement and isolation of the head fragment and fractures with comminution of the head fragment). But the majority of patients with 4-part fractures do not receive a prosthesis.

*Lettin:* Dr. Watson states it is possible to convert to an arthrodesis after a failed total arthroplasty. I would like to ask him how often he has tried this. I am interested to know, because these cases are absent from the published series, and because all the reoperated patients received a new prosthesis.

*Watson:* That is correct. The series we reported on did not include revisions of Neer prostheses. But while I was working with Dr. Neer, there were several cases in which we removed other types of prosthesis and tried arthrodeses. I remember one case where that was particularly difficult. That patient also had an infection, so we first removed the prosthesis and performed a debridement. Then we performed an arthrodesis in a second sitting. I personally have removed the prosthesis in uninfected cases and have had good results with the ASIF technique, which is very stable. When it is necessary to avoid using that much metal, as in cases of infection, we have tried approximating the humerus to the glenoid, inserting bone grafts, and immobilizing the shoulder for several months. That is a difficult approach, and the success rate is not very high. We have also used this technique in uninfected cases. We treated three patients in this way, and I believe that all went on to bony union. I operated another case only 4 months ago, and the outcome is not yet definite, although healing seems to be progressing well.

# On the Treatment of Comminuted Fracture-Dislocations of the Proximal Humerus: Internal Fixation or Prosthetic Replacement

R. Marti, T.E. Lim, C.W. Jolles

## Introduction

Approximately 85% of proximal humeral fractures are minimally displaced, impacted, and therefore stable on motion. The functional outcome in these cases is affected little by minor amounts of angulation and lateral displacement. These fractures, which are most commonly seen in 60- to 70-year-olds, can be satisfactorily managed with early functional exercises. The remaining 15% of proximal humeral fractures are a challenge to diagnosis and treatment - to diagnosis, because the displacement is difficult to assess on standard radiographs; and to treatment, because the prognosis relates closely to the initial displacement. One problem is that comminuted fracture-dislocations can rarely be reduced stably enough to allow functional rehabilitation; another is that there is a significant risk of later avascular necrosis of the humeral head. The average age of this group is somewhat younger, at about 60 years. Traditional classifications of fractures like those described by Kocher (1896) and later by Böhler take into account only mechanical and morphologic aspects. Today, however, when prosthetic treatments have become a reality, the vascular and biologic aspects of fractures have an important bearing on the type of treatment selected.

The Neer classification (1970) takes into account both the morphologic and the prognostic aspects of proximal humeral fractures. It is based on the number of fracture fragments and their displacement (Fig. 1).

Minimally displaced fractures present similar therapeutic and prognostic problems, regardless of the number of fracture lines. Their prevalence among proximal humeral fractures is 85%, and the great majority are amenable to functional treatment. Displaced fractures should be very carefully analyzed with regard to their displacement and associated joint incongruity, and with regard to the possibility of avascular necrosis. A four-part fracture with avulsion of both tuberosities and an isolated head fragment causes the most severe compromise of blood supply to the humeral head. A large head fragment that is undislocated is not at serious risk for avascular necrosis.

The incidence of avascular necrosis increases with the degree of displacement and is extremely high in four-part fracture-dislocations.

Here we shall focus our attention on these problem fractures, i.e., comminuted fractures and fracture-dislocations of the proximal humerus (Neer IV-VI). In addition to following operatively treated fractures prospectively, we conducted a retrospective review of nine conservatively treated cases for purposes of comparison.

Shoulder Replacement
Eds.: Kölbel/Helbig/Blauth

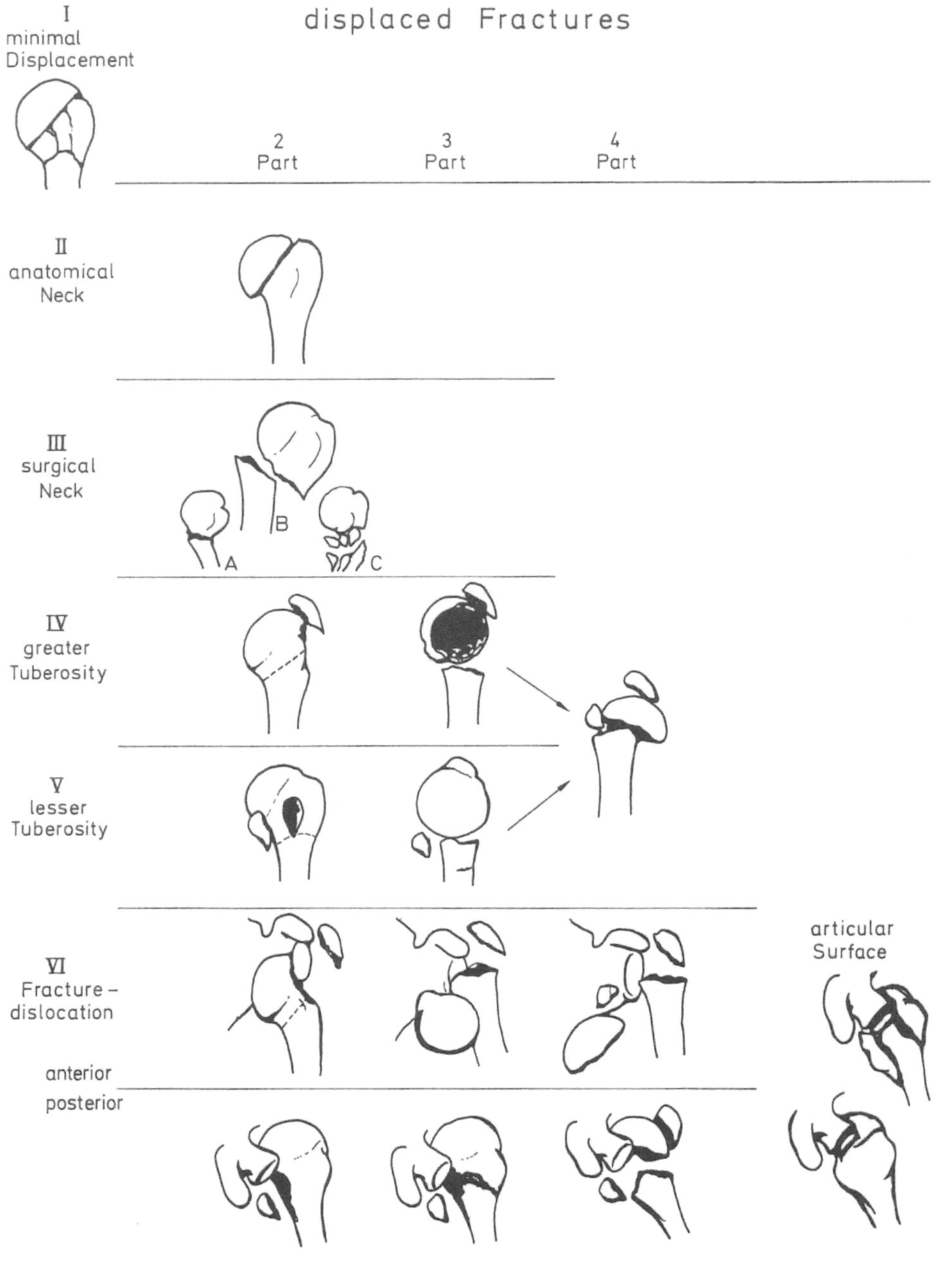


**Fig. 1.** The Neer classification of proximal humeral fractures

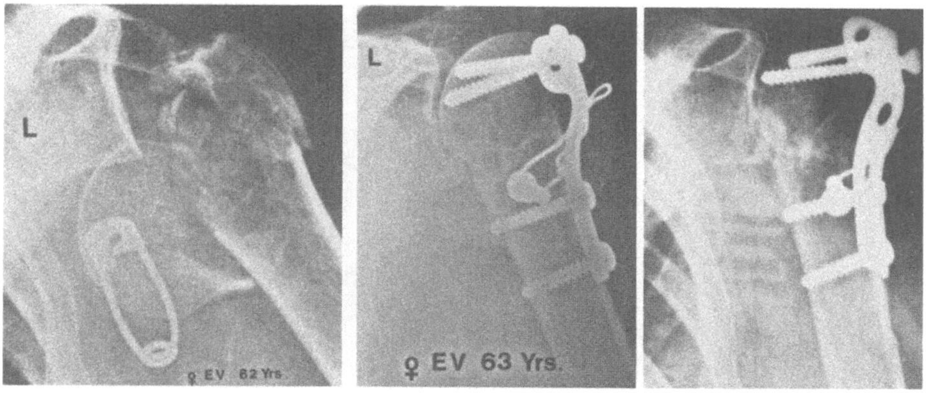


**Fig. 2.** Comminuted fracture-dislocation treated by internal plating. Extensive avascular necrosis, poor result

## Therapeutic Guidelines

Minimally displaced three- and four-part fractures are treated with early functional exercise. In fractures that become displaced secondarily, the same principles are followed as for primarily displaced fractures.

Basically two surgical options are available: *internal fixation* and *prosthetic replacement.*

With *internal fixation,* care is taken not to cause further damage to the blood supply of the humeral head (Fig. 2) [3]. Like other authors, we have obtained good results with open reduction and minimal internal fixation [1, 4, 5]. The head fragment can be fixed in impaction by wiring the individual fragments to the humeral shaft (Figs. 3-5). Lag screws can also be placed to improve the potential for revascularization. It is unnecessary to open the capsule, even in fracture-dislocations, as this might compromise the residual blood supply (Fig. 4). Any valgus impaction of the head should be left uncorrected for similar reasons. The stability obtained is sufficient for early postoperative functional treatment and contributes to revascularization.

Thus, the treatment of comminuted fractures of the proximal humerus is guided by the potential for avascular necrosis. Displaced fractures in which the head fragment is not dislocated can be treated by minimal internal fixation with wire loops.

The same applies to fracture-dislocations in younger individuals.

## Results

In 1983 we reported on 21 patients, 9 of whom were treated conservatively, 9 by internal fixation, and 3 with a prosthesis [4]. In late 1985 and early 1986 we reviewed comminuted fractures and fracture-dislocations of the proximal humerus (Neer IV and VI) that we had treated operatively between 1974 and 1984. This series of 24 patients had 13 comminuted fractures without dislocation of the head, and 11 comminuted fracture-dislocations. Nineteen were treated by internal fixation, and 5 were treated primarily with a Neer prosthesis. The average age of the patients was 63 years. Fifteen of the 19 internal fixations were done with tension-band wires, and 4 were done with a plate.

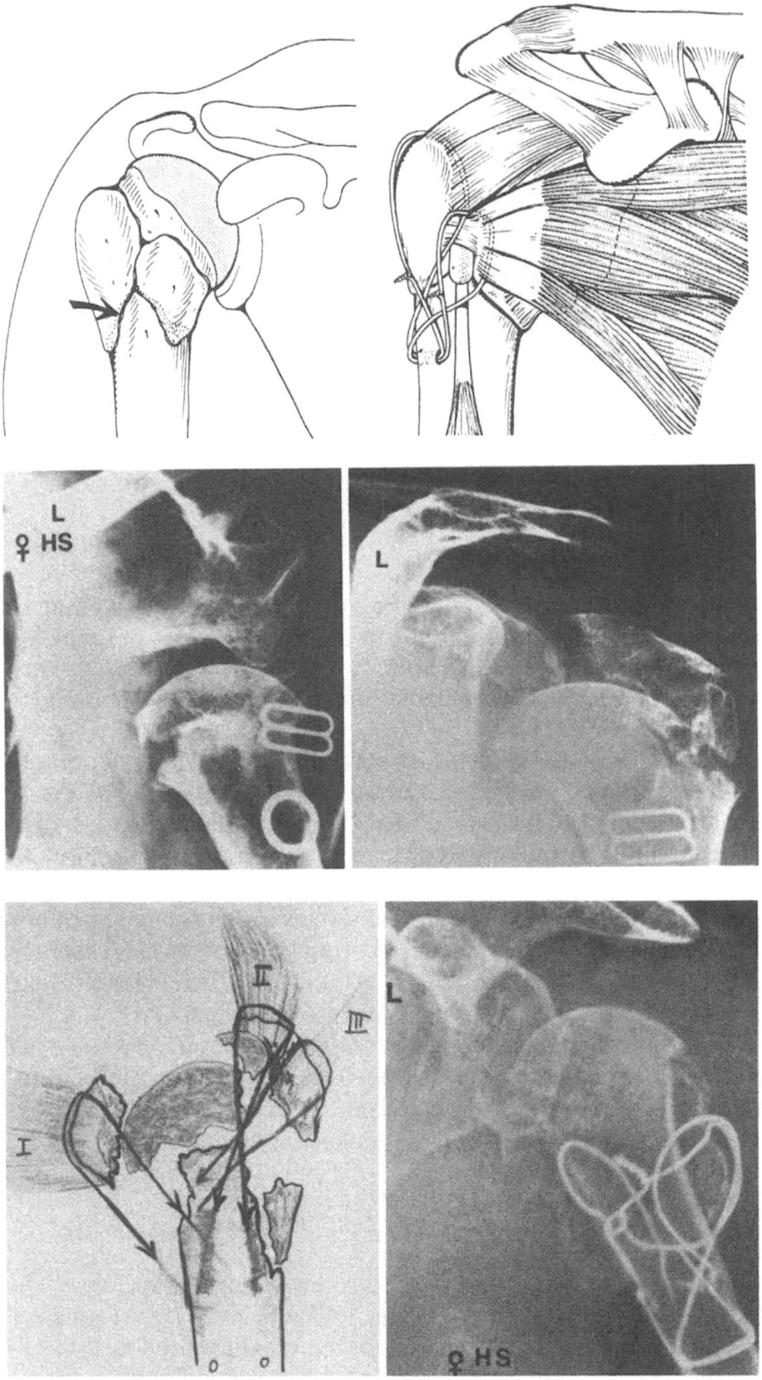


a

b

**Fig. 3a.** Minimal internal fixation by the tension-band principle involves wiring the individual components of the rotator cuff and corresponding bone fragments to the humeral shaft, which is impacted into the head. **b** One to three wire loops are used, depending on the number of fracture fragments. It may be best to fix the supra- and infraspinatus separately. **c** The example shows a comminuted fracture-dislocation with interposed fragments after reduction. The fracture has been stably fixed with three wire loops functioning as tension bands

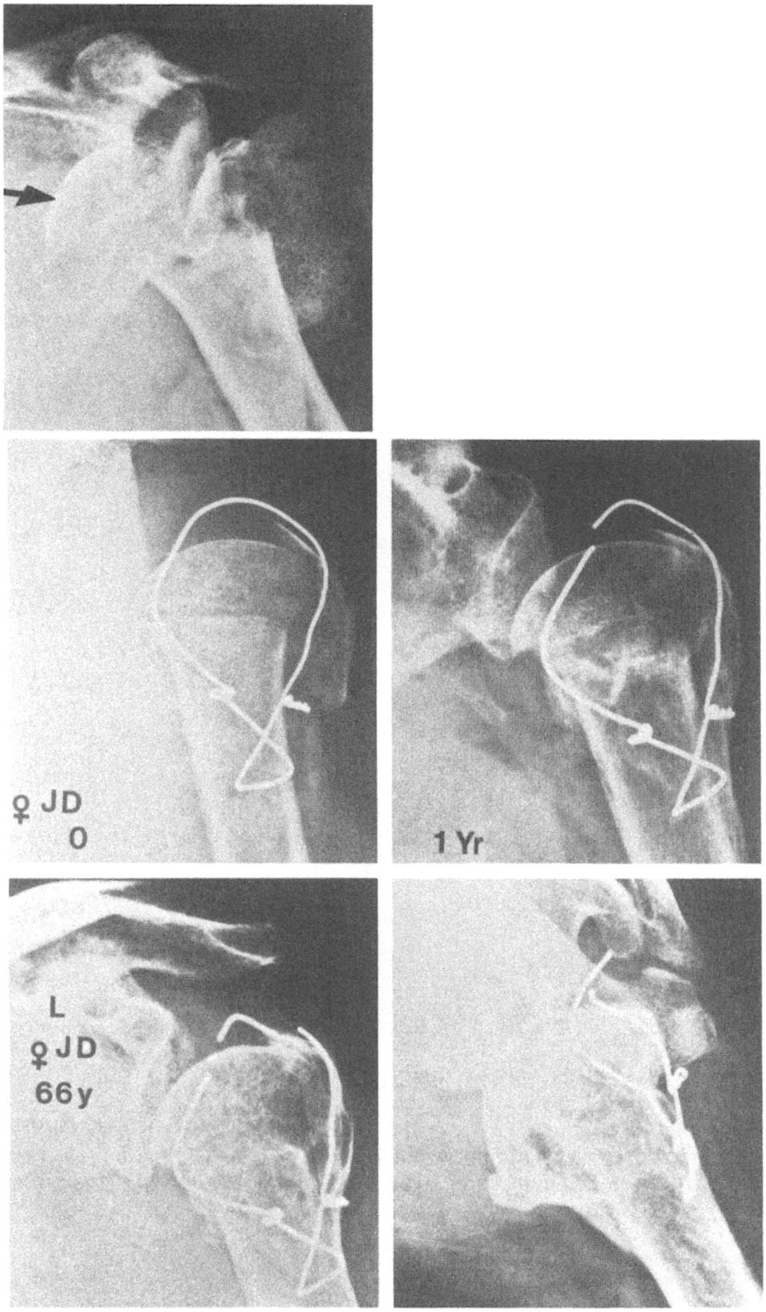


**Fig. 4.** Comminuted fracture with a markedly displaced head fragment *(arrow)* treated by simple tension-band wiring. The low-lying head is reduced by muscular traction during healing. After 5 years the head is revascularized and shows no deformity

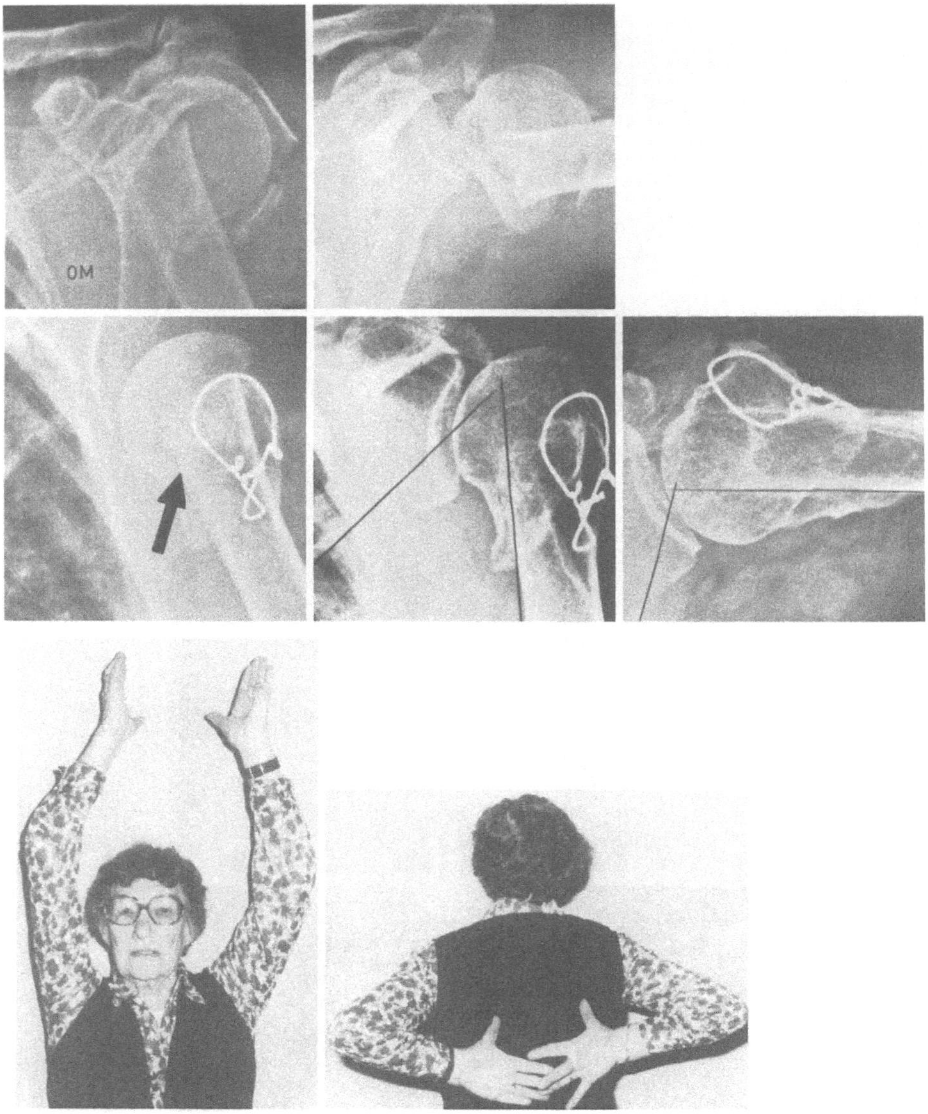


a

b

**Fig. 5 a.** Irreducible comminuted fracture 4 weeks after conservative therapy. Simple tension-band fixation with impaction of the shaft into the large head fragment *(arrow)*. **b** Eight years later the head is perfectly positioned in the joint. The patient is pain-free and has almost symmetrical function

At follow-up, 19 of the 24 patients were satisfied with the result – 4 of the 5 fracture-dislocations treated with a prosthesis, and 15 of the 19 patients treated by internal fixation. One-fourth of the results were rated good according to the objective criteria of Neer, and three-fourths were rated as fair to poor. It is noteworthy that poor ratings were given to four of the five cases treated with a prosthesis.

Marked avascular necrosis of the humeral head was diagnosed in 11 of the 19 fractures managed by internal fixation. Only four of these patients had com-

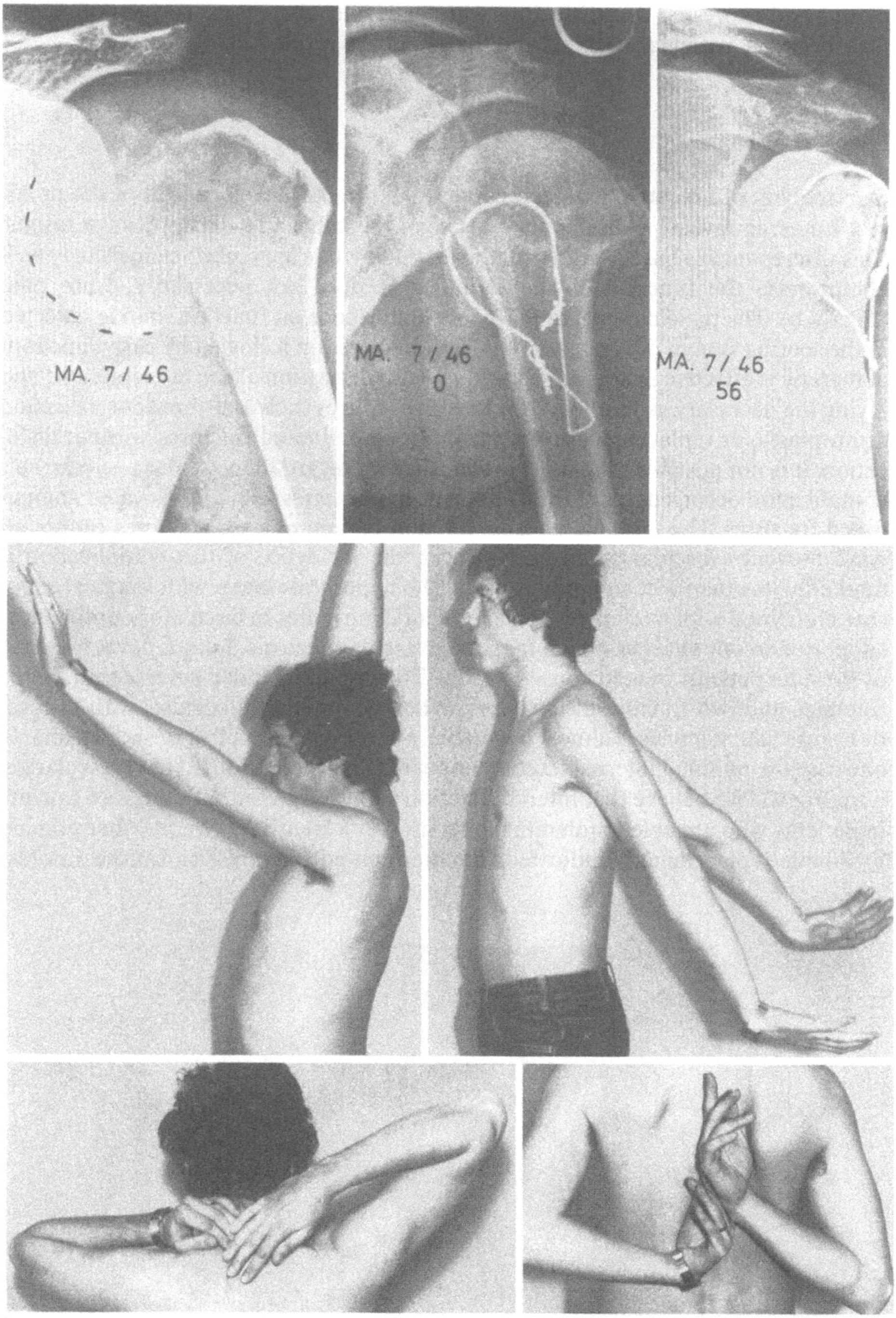


a

b

**Fig. 6a.** Old comminuted fracture-dislocation. Marked avascular necrosis is apparent 1 year after fixation with a tension band. **b** Ten years postoperatively shoulder motion is restricted, but the patient is fully able to work and has only mild complaints. To date this young patient has not been reoperated plaints and expressed dissatisfaction with the result. There is no correlation, therefore, between avascular necrosis and the subjective result.

## Discussion

Our analysis of operatively treated comminuted fracture-dislocations of the proximal humerus reveals a discrepancy between the subjective and objective results. This discrepancy is based largely on the fact that while avascular necrosis may well compromise the function of the shoulder, it does not necessarily cause pain (Fig. 6 a,b). The patients seem to place less importance on function than is reflected in the scoring system of Neer. Minimal internal fixation followed by early functional therapy is effective in achieving partial revascularization of the humeral head and laying the necessary groundwork for later procedures such as arthrodesis, resection arthroplasty, or replacement arthroplasty. In comminuted fractures without dislocation, it is not possible to make a prognosis with regard to avascular necrosis; this complication occurred in 6 of the 13 patients in our series with undislocated comminuted fractures. The minimal internal fixation of comminuted fractures cannot always prevent avascular necrosis. However, the incidence of this complication is markedly less than when plating is used. The hypothesis that a wide surgical exposure combined with a relatively large implant contributes to circulatory problems is supported in our analysis by the fact that avascular necrosis did not develop in any of the nine patients treated conservatively. This group included seven comminuted fractures and two fracture-dislocations. When comminution coexists with dislocation, avascular necrosis is almost inevitable. We observed it in five of six patients. In one case the minimal internal fixation appears to have contributed to revascularization (Fig. 4). We believe that internal fixation is preferred for both types of fracture in patients who are able to tolerate reoperation at a later time. We feel that primary prosthetic replacement is indicated for comminuted fracture-dislocations in older

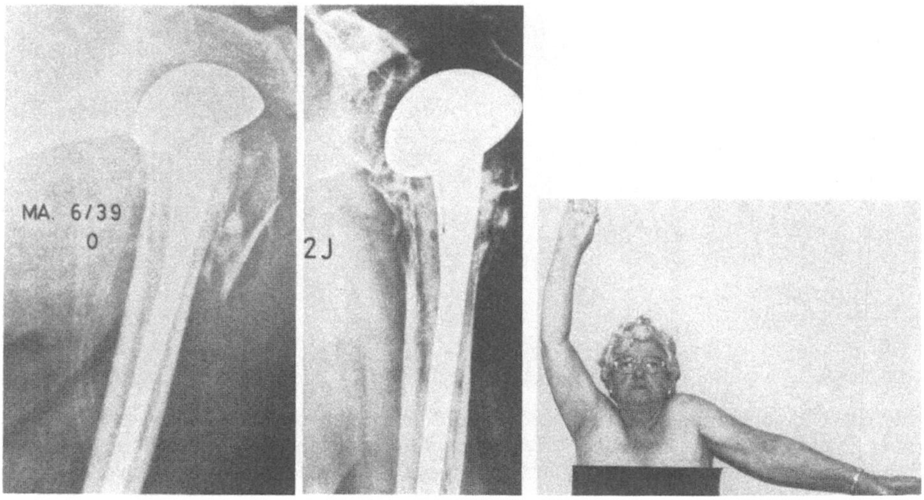


**Fig. 7.** Primary Neer prosthesis. The patient has no significant complaints, but the result corresponds to an arthrodesis (see Fig. 9)

patients with preexisting disability. Comminution without dislocation is considered a relative indication in older patients. The operating team should be prepared for both procedures. The deltopectoral approach is recommended as a good general-purpose approach. The same tension-band wires can be used to reconstruct the rotator cuff when a primary prosthesis is inserted; the approach is the same.

## Secondary Procedures

Nonunions are rare in both operatively and conservatively treated cases [6]. Patients complain of severe pain, limited motion, and loss of strength.

Given the poorly perfused and sclerosed condition of the bone ends, absolute stability can be achieved only by internal plating, possibly combined with a tension band (Fig. 7). Bone grafting contributes to rapid union. The procedure is worth-

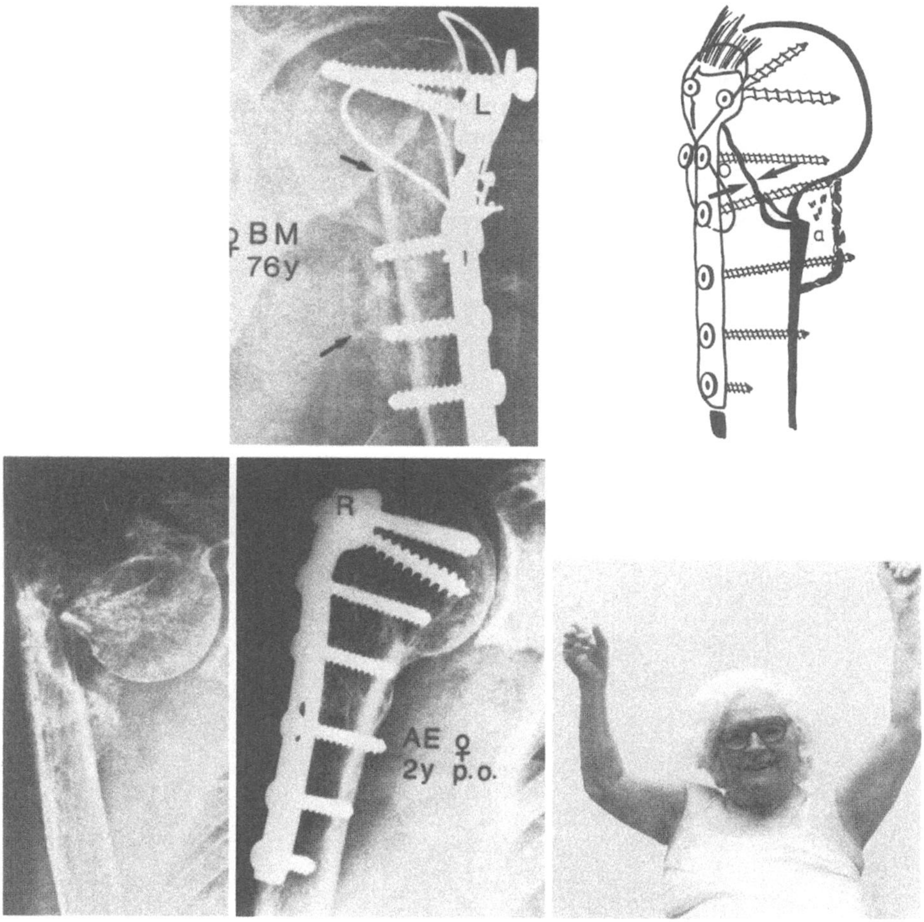


**Fig. 8 a.** Nonunions are treated by stabilizing the site with a plate, tension band, and a medial free cancellous bone graft. **b** with adequate screw purchase in the humeral head, it is sufficient to impact the shaft fragment into the head and apply a plate. Postoperatively there is excellent consolidation with pain relief and acceptable function while even in the elderly, and shoulder motion is gradually regained (Fig. 8 a,b). The tension band gives the screws a more secure hold in the proximal humerus. All seven of the nonunions in our series went on to union when this type of internal fixation was used. The patients were free of complaints and had acceptable strength with an average abduction of 130° - this with an average age of 65 years (29-82). Arthrodesis presents no technical problems in cases where avascular necrosis has occurred. Because of the compromised condition of the bone, we recommend bridging the site with a plate according to standard ASIF technique; this may be combined with an autologous bone graft if necessary (Fig. 9). Arthrodesis is far more difficult after a failed replacement arthroplasty, and extensive bone grafting is needed for a successful result (Fig. 10 a-c).

Resection arthroplasty can lead to a satisfying functional result, provided the rotator cuff is reattached on osteotomized fragments of bone. We have had no experience to date with total shoulder replacement arthroplasty.

## Summary

The end result of a proximal humeral fracture relates directly to the original configuration of the fracture. The Neer system meets essential requirements for classifying these types of injury. The operating technique and choice of implant affect the inci-

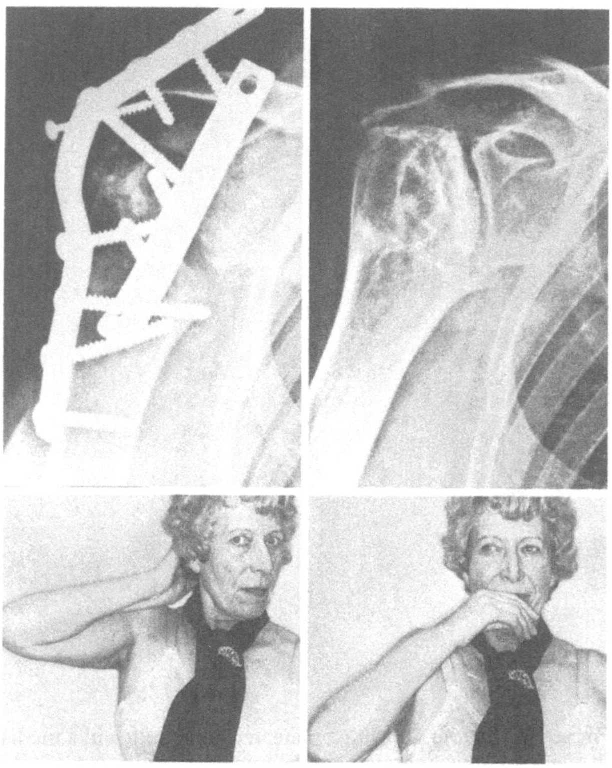

**Fig. 9.** Avascular necrosis following conservative treatment of a fracture. Arthrodesis with a plate led to an acceptable functional result

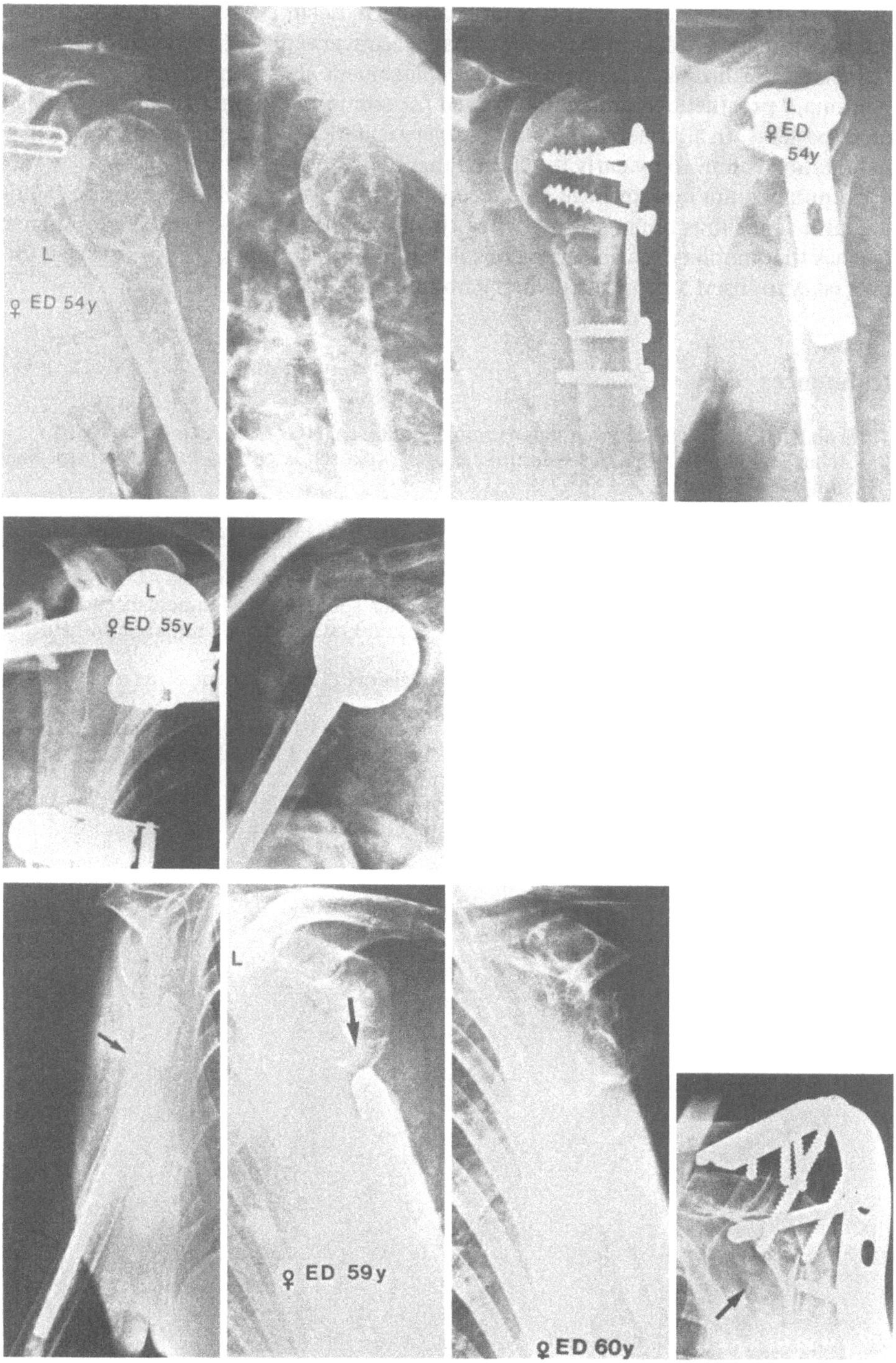


**Fig. 10 a.** Four-part fracture was initially treated by improper plate fixation. **b** Insertion of a cemented prosthesis was followed by dislocation and severe pain. **c** The prosthesis could not be removed, and so the head was sawed off, resulting in a painful flail arm. The patient was referred to our center. **c** In an initial operation the stem of the prosthesis was removed, and later we performed a bridging arthrodesis using a plate and corticocancellous grafts. This case illustrates the problem of plate fixation, secondary prosthetic replacement, and the difficulty of arthrodesis following prosthetic treatment dence of avascular necrosis. This complication can occur even years after the injury but may remain asymptomatic as far as pain is concerned. Later procedures such as arthrodesis, arthroplasty, and prosthetic replacement are still possible.

Primary prosthetic treatment is reserved for comminuted fracture-dislocations in older patients. In all other cases where surgery is indicated, we prefer minimal internal fixation followed by early functional therapy.

Nonunions are rare and can be successfully managed by plating, tension banding, and cancellous bone grafting when the humeral head is viable [6]. Experience teaches that mobility returns after consolidation of the nonunion; this makes it unnecessary to insert a prosthesis when a nonunion is diagnosed.

## References

1. Jakob RP, Ganz R (1981) Proximale Humerusfrakturen. Helv Chir Acta 48: 595-610
2. Kocher T (1896) Beiträge zur Kenntnis einiger praktisch wichtiger Frakturformen. Sallmann, Basel Leipzig
3. Laing PG (1956) The arterial supply of the adult humerus. J Bone Joint Surg [Am] 38: 1105
4. Lim TE, Ochsner PE, Marti R, Holscher AA (1983) The results of treatment of comminuted fractures and fracture dislocations of the proximal humerus. Neth J Surg 35/4
5. Magerl F (1974) Osteosynthesen im Bereich der Schulter. Helv Chir Acta 41: 225
6. Marti R, Ochsner PE, Lim TE (1984) Therapie der subkapitalen Humeruspseudarthrose. In: Chapchall G (Hrsg) Verletzungen und Erkrankungen der Schulterregion. Thieme, Stuttgart New York
7. Müller ME, Allgöwer M, Schneider R, Willenegger H (1979) Manual of internal fixation. Springer, Berlin Heidelberg New York
8. Neer CS (1970) Displaced proximal humerus fractures (I). J Bone Joint Surg [Am] 52: 1077
9. Neer CS (1970) Displaced proximal humerus fractures (II). J Bone Joint Surg [Am] 52: 1090

## Discussion

*Watson:* Your paper brought out several points that are not inconsistent with our policies. There are many points on which we agree.

Apparently there are some cases in which avascular necrosis will not occur. In these cases, when the patient is older and does not expect too much in the way of functional recovery, both treatment methods will give acceptable results.

I believe that it is very important to reconstruct, and when we do this, we perform internal fixations more often than we insert prostheses. Although many of the cases shown had bad fractures, most are not really so severe, and the majority - perhaps 80% - do not require surgery at all. But if there are marked displacements of the fragments, I think that they should be reduced and fixed.

Because I personally have had a great deal of experience with the prosthesis and postoperative rehabilitation, I believe that I can do more for my patients in some situations with prosthetic reconstruction than with internal fixation. Someone with Dr. Marti's experience with internal fixations may be in the opposite situation, and I can appreciate that internal fixation might be of greater benefit.

Wire breakage has caused us serious concern, mainly because of the danger of wire fragments getting into the joint. Apparently the problem is different from in the hip, where trochanteric wires often break and may or may not cause problems but rarely migrate into the joint. It has been our impression that the shoulder literally attracts such wire fragments, and we have often had to remove metal on this account. I would be interested to know what Dr. Marti thinks about this.

*Marti:* As far as wire breakage is concerned, we have seen instances of it, but the fragments were not a problem because they remained in the soft tissues. An alternative would be to fix fragments to the humeral shaft with nylon or dacron, as we use for ligament reconstructions.

*Blauth:* Doesn't the small number of cases make it difficult for you to draw conclusions?

*Marti:* Fracture-dislocations are not common, and in view of this, 31 cases are not a small number. Typically this is an injury of the eldery. But I have shown you a man 26 years of age, another man 36, and a woman 52, and we should talk about the indications in these patients.

With regard to patients over 65 years of age, I have come to the conclusion that we should no longer be so ambitious with internal fixations as we were in the past, and that prosthetic replacement would be a better option.

(Editor's note: Contrasts of viewpoints are very apparent. Dr. Watson considers prosthetic replacement a technically demanding procedure that requires intensive, prolonged rehabilitation. But prosthetic arthroplasty appears to be safe and effective even on a long-term basis, and the functional results are superior. This is the rationale for using prostheses even in relatively young individuals. Dr. Marti considers reconstruction by internal fixation more demanding and apparently considers the "insertion of a prosthesis" less demanding for the treatment of fractures. He also appears to have less confidence in the long-term success of a prosthesis. Thus, a trend is emerging that is analogous to the hip joint - the tendency to favor internal fixation with preservation of the joint in younger patients, and prosthetic replacement in older patients.)

*Chairman:* I gather from the reports of Dr. Watson and Dr. Cofield that patients in the United States probably place somewhat higher demands on treatment than in Europe, and that this is a major reason why the cutoff age has been lowered in candidates for replacement arthroplasty. While we have by no means exhausted the topic of proximal humeral fracture therapy, we have had an opportunity to discuss the limited role of prosthetic replacement in the management of these fractures.

# Polyacetal Resin Shoulder Prostheses for Posttraumatic Conditions and Osteoarthritis

C. Burri

Today there is no question that properly designed shoulder prostheses, like the polyacetal resin device of Mathys, have earned an established place in the treatment of tumors of the proximal humerus that require a segmental resection of bone. In these cases the insertion of a tumor prosthesis offers a real alternative to disarticulation. The use of autologous grafts (e.g., fibular transplantation), with or without microvascular attachment, aroused much interest initially but is becoming less prominent because of the inability to restore joint congruity, and because of the favorable results and zero incidence of secondary degeneration that have occurred with the isoelastic polyacetal resin prosthesis. We have extremely satisfying clinical observations dating back more than 12 years. With this type of prosthesis there appears to be no danger of stem loosening after the first 6–12 months, and the longevity of the implant appears to be excellent owing to the intimate contact that exists between the stem and bone. Our investigations of two postmortem specimens confirmed the strength of the prosthesis and its anchorage, and biomechanical measurements at various sites along the prosthetic stem have enabled us to make additional design improvements.

The prosthesis appears to have a more limited indication for osteoarthritic conditions of the shoulder, in which we are dealing less with radiologic changes than with the subjective and objective status of the individual. A good candidate is the patient with rheumatoid arthritis who must use his arm for support because of general infirmity. We also consider the prosthesis in patients with posttraumatic conditions such as avascular necrosis, traumatic arthritis, and nonunions that cause significant, painful limitation of shoulder mobility.

Two main types of prosthesis are available for these indications – a simple humeral head prosthesis which comes in various head and stem diameters, and a spherical prosthesis that performs only a supportive function and is reserved for the rare cases where the humeral head is lost and the rotator insertions are absent (Figs. 1 a-d, 2 a,b). We have inserted a total prosthesis in only two cases. Glenoid loosening with secondary dislocation occurred in one patient and necessitated removal of the glenoid component. We have come to regard polyacetal resin as an extremely tissue-compatible material, and we have seen no instances of painful secondary degeneration in more than 10 years' experience when the correct head size is used. The fact that the shoulder is subjected to relatively low mechanical stresses supports this conclusion.

## Operative Technique

The necessary head diameter, stem length and caliber of the prosthesis can be determined with a plastic overlay placed on the radiograph of the affected or contralateral shoulder. The patient is positioned supine with the arm draped free for mobility.

Shoulder Replacement
Eds.: Kölbel/Helbig/Blauth

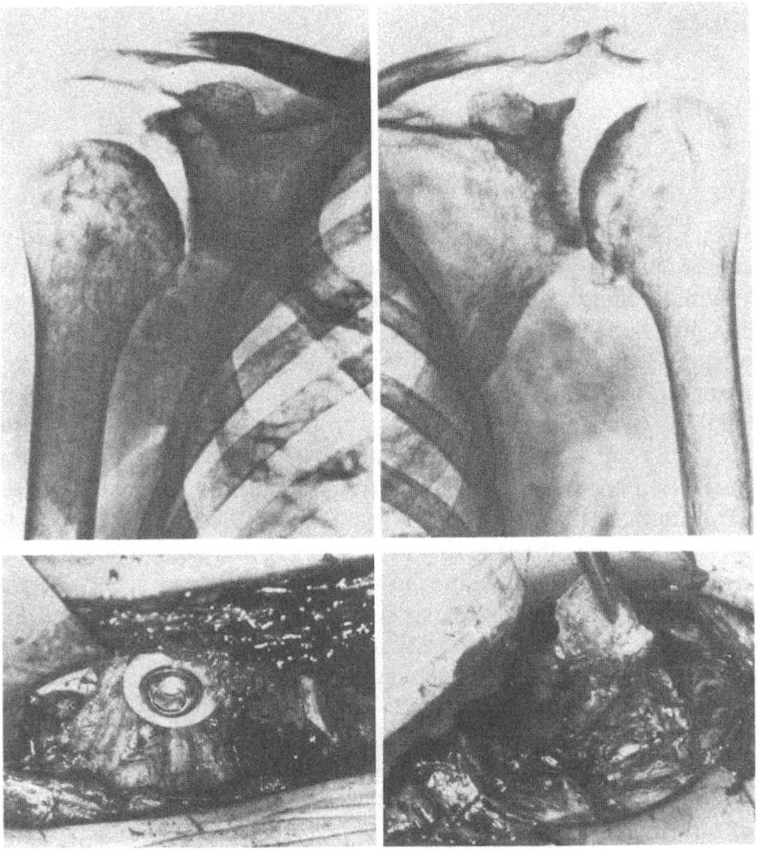

a

b

**Fig. 1 a-d.** Bilateral prostheses in a patient with osteoarthritis of both shoulders. **a** Preoperative radiographs. **b** Operative photos: The insertion of the subscapularis, osteotomized for placement of the prosthesis, is reattached with a screw and washer. **c** Follow-up radiographs. **d** Functional result

The skin incision starts proximally over the acromion and curves distally over the deltopectoral groove. The landmark is the cephalic vein, and the deep approach is made at its lateral border. The anterior origin of the deltoid is incised if necessary, and the subscapularis muscle is exposed. Anatomic orientation may be difficult in patients with a comminuted fracture-dislocation, but in all cases one should identify the rotator and subscapularis insertions and preserve their continuity with the corresponding tendon or tendinous expansion. In osteoarthritics and rheumatoids, our latest technique is to osteotomize just the insertion of the subscapularis and excise the capsule.

Even without osteotomy of the coracoid, an excellent view of the shoulder joint is obtained. In comminuted cases an attempt should always be made to reattach the tendinous insertions directly to the prosthesis in their original positions. We feel it is extremely important in such cases to establish bony continuity with the humeral shaft. Only this can guarantee good mobility and longevity of the reconstruction.

After removing the head fragment or after resecting the altered head, we use a medullary reamer to prepare the humeral shaft for insertion of the prosthesis. The

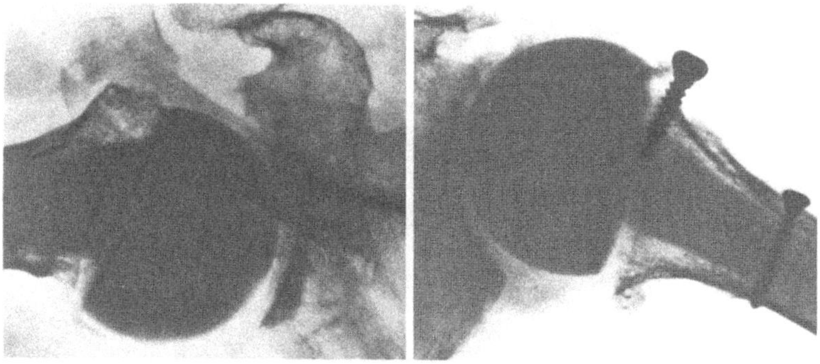

c

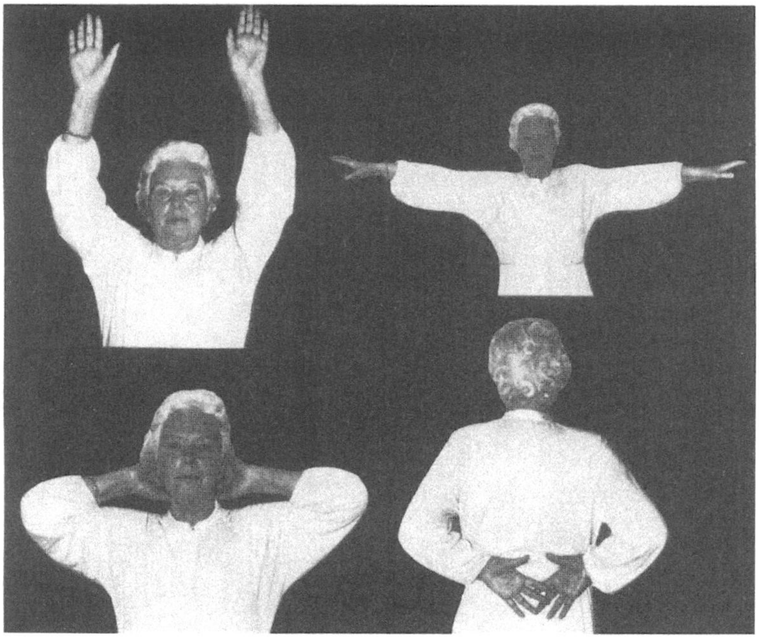

d

**Fig. 1 c and d.**

standard medullary reaming instrument of the ASIF has proved better for this purpose than the special hand reamers, because increments of 0.5 mm are possible with the power reamer. There is a danger, of course, that the flexible reamer shaft will cut a slightly S-shaped cavity, but the stem of the prosthesis can adapt to this adequately. A conical reamer is used to shape the upper end of the humerus for a press fit. Once the humerus has been prepared to receive the selected stem, the head prosthesis is inserted in 40° of retroversion. This increased retrotilt corresponds to the angle that Weber aims for in his derotation osteotomy and is an effective safeguard against dislocation. The oblique seating of the prosthesis against the bone end and the ridged neck of the prosthesis afford adequate rotational stability. However, we recommend the placement of a separate anchoring screw as an added precaution. For this purpose we use a small-fragment cortex screw inserted through the humerus and prosthetic stem 3–5 cm distal to the bone end. Cement is not used.

In simple osteoarthritis, the osteotomized bone fragment with the subcaspularis insertion is fitted into the defect and attached to the prosthesis with a screw, making

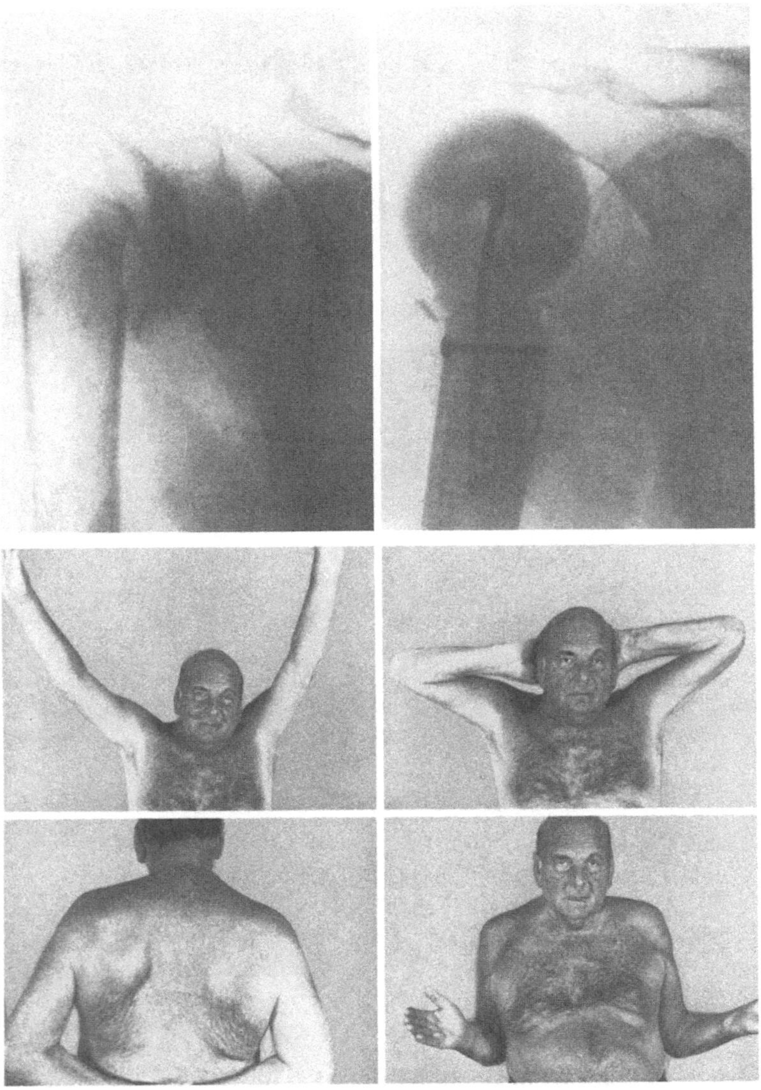

a b

**Fig. 2 a,b.** Painless nonunion of the humeral head with very severe limitation of function. **a** Radiographs before and after insertion of a spherical-head prosthesis. **b** Functional result

sure to establish contact between the resected edges so that bony consolidation can occur.

In comminuted cases the tendinous insertions are likewise attached to the prosthesis at their physiologic sites, and residual defects are packed with autologous cancellous bone (e.g., from the resected part of the humeral head) to restore osseous continuity in the proximal humerus. This phase of the procedure is more difficult when the entire humeral head is lost and the rotator cuff can no longer be defined (see Fig. 2). Here there is no recourse other than to anchor a spherical prosthesis firmly in the shaft, reduce the shoulder, and close the wound in layers over a pair of suction drains, one deep and one superficial.

The arm is placed on an abduction splint postoperatively. The splint is removed as soon as the patient is able to perform active assisted exercises from the splint without pain. If the patient is able to raise the arm above the horizontal without assistance, splinting may be omitted. The technique involving reattachment of severed or avulsed tendon insertions has yielded a marked improvement of results compared with the multicentric study concluded in 1975.

Below we shall present follow-up results for 60 patients who were treated with an isoelastic shoulder prosthesis for the indications stated above.

## Results

To the collaborative study from 30 hospitals we added our own most recent cases, making a total of 166 implanted shoulder prostheses - 35 for acute trauma, 63 for osteoarthritis and posttraumatic conditions, and 68 for neoplasms.

Sixty patients (26 men, 34 women) with an average age of 52.4 years (32-78 years) were followed an average of 37 months after placement of the prosthesis.

*Technique:* In the great majority of cases (53) the incision was made in the deltopectoral groove. Acromion osteotomy (7 patients) was occasionally used in the past but is no longer practiced today. Forty-seven of the patients received the standard humeral prosthesis, 10 the spherical-head prosthesis, 1 a tumor prosthesis, and 2 a total shoulder prosthesis. Today we believe that the standard humeral prosthesis should be used whenever possible, combining it with a resection angle of 45°.

The prosthesis was attached without screws in 3 cases, with 1 screw in 50 cases, with 2 screws in 5, and with cement in 2 cases from the original study.

The technique of muscular reattachment also has changed since the original study, and today screw fixation is our method of choice. Overall, sutures were used in 18 cases, and biceps duplication in 2 cases; reattachment could not be obtained in 5 cases.

As mentioned earlier, we prefer to position the arm in abduction for a brief period after surgery. We no longer use traction or the Desault bandage.

Complications consisted of 4 hematomas, 2 infections, 2 cases of loosening, 2 cases of early prosthetic fracture, and 3 dislocations.

Nineteen patients rated the subjective result as excellent, 27 as good, 10 as fair, and only 4 as poor. Thirty-one patients reported no complaints, 18 reported occasional complaints, 5 had frequent complaints, and 6 described their complaints as severe.

We may say, then, that the isoelastic shoulder prosthesis gives favorable subjective results in more than 80% of cases. Range of motion - the major criterion for evaluating success in posttraumatic shoulders - was markedly better than in the earlier series owing to the use of screws for tendon reattachment. On average the patients had 95° of anterior elevation, 87° of lateral elevation, 54° of internal rotation, and 36° of external rotation. It should be added that nine patients suffered from posttraumatic nerve damage, mainly involving the axillary nerve, which can have a significant impact on total range of motion.

An increased range of motion was obtained in 56-59 of the 60 patients reviewed.

Very few patients recover an absolutely complete range of shoulder motion with the isoelastic prosthesis. But in many cases the limitation is small enough that it does not produce significant disability in normal daily activities.

The most outstanding technical innovation of recent years has been the effort to fix, where possible, the rotator tendon insertions to the isoelastic shoulder prosthesis in a stable fashion. Anchoring the tendon attachments to the prosthesis with screws in a way that creates osseous continuity with the residual bone of the proximal humerus, using grafted autologous bone as necessary, had led to a significant improvement of results. We feel that the polyacetal resin prosthesis, when used in the correct size and design and with appropriate instrumentation, has earned an established place in the treatment of posttraumatic lesions of the shoulder.

## Summary

The major indication for the isoelastic shoulder prosthesis is in tumor surgery where prosthetic replacement is compatible with the priority demand for adequate surgical margins. Use of the prosthesis also may be considered in rheumatoid patients and patients with significant disability after trauma (especially fracture-dislocations). With the prosthesis made of polyacetal resin, it is possible to reattach the tendon insertions to the implant with screws - an option not available in metallic prostheses. The functional results depend largely on the ability to reconstruct the soft tissues, especially the rotators. Complications are infrequent with proper technique, and the cementless fixation of the isoelastic prosthesis provides a solid, permanent anchorage in nearly all cases. Heterotopic calcifications is believed to pose the greatest potential threat to long-term results.

## References

Burri C, Rüter A (1977) Prothesen und Alternativen am Arm, Teil I: Schultergelenk. Huber, Bern Stuttgart Wien

## Discussion

*Chairman:* You stated that the average follow-up was 14 months. I would be interested to know when the last follow-up examination was performed in this group.

*Burri:* We published this series in 1974. There are hardly any cases that were reexamined since that time, and we have started follow-ups for our own patients.

*Chairman:* Have you had any problems with drill holes placed at the junction of the head and neck of the prosthesis?

*Burri:* No, we have not seen any fractures through the screw holes.

*Chairman:* You showed one case of nonunion. Can you tell us something more about this indication?

*Burri:* In the case you refer to, the head fragment was in very poor condition. Nonunions are not uncommon after subcapital humeral fractures. We have found 24 cases, 8 in our own patients. Motion at the nonunion is very pronounced, and stabilizing the bone restores shoulder movement and alleviates stiffness. It was not my intention, though, to present my position on fractures or nonunions, but only to describe the use of the shoulder prosthesis in selected cases.

*Thomas:* You reattach the rotator cuff insertions with screws at the initial operation. How does this contribute to definitive healing and long-term function of the rotator cuff?

*Burri:* The screw simply holds the fragment with the rotators against the shaft, so that it stays in place. The cancellous bone grafts provide for long-term stability.

*Chairman:* Reattachment of the tuberosities is also done with the Neer prosthesis, and often the tuberosities are reconstructed with cancellous bone harvested from the iliac crest. Resorption is a frequent problem in these cases. Have you seen a similar phenomenon when you reattach the tuberosities?

*Burri:* When autologous tissue is interposed, we know from hip surgery that it takes 6-8 weeks for an autologous graft to become solid. During this time we must avoid stressing the site and use continuous passive motion in preference to active exercises that might dislodge the grafts.

*Gekeler:* How much wear is the polyacetal prosthesis subject to during function?

*Burri:* We have abandoned trials with total prostheses because we were dissatisfied with the glenoid. But we have seen cases at 12-14 years that look practically the same as they did at 1 year. I will return to this point later in connection with tumors, where I have a slide showing the joint cartilage 18 months after hemiarthroplasty.

*Lettin:* One of the most interesting things brought to light by the discussion is that Prof. Marti (internal fixation) and Prof. Burri (prosthetic replacement) had virtually the same results as far as range of motion is concerned. It has been my experience that one cannot expect arm elevation above shoulder level, except perhaps with the Neer prosthesis. Prof. Burri's results with rotational motion were of course very good.

Again, this supports my contention that our results may to a certain extent be "preordained," much as they are in fractures of the femoral neck. Whatever technique we use, we know that there will be a certain incidence of avascular necrosis, and that shoulders will tend to develop posttraumatic adhesions. We must expect some limitation of motion, therefore.

I consider it significant that the 10 patients of Prof. Marti treated with a Neer prosthesis were able to raise their arm only to about 90°, but that all were pain-free. Their range of motion actually was no better than with an arthrodesis. But I believe that the insertion of a humeral prosthesis is a simpler operation than arthrodesis, and that it requires less postoperative immobilization. So, the operation is definitely worthwhile despite the limited range of motion.

# Shoulder Replacement: Prognosis Related to Diagnosis

R. H. Cofield

Pain relief after total shoulder replacement is generally acceptable for all diagnostic groups. However, motion and strength may vary from one diagnostic category to the next, as may the nature and frequency of complications.

## Osteoarthritis

The pathologic features of osteoarthritis are fairly standard. The bone is sclerotic, the humeral head is flattened centrally and to some extent superiorly, there are peripheral osteophytes, the glenoid is flattened and often shows posterior erosion, the anterior capsule is tight, rotator cuff tears are infrequent, and there is a tendency for posterior humeral subluxation (Fig. 1). Three series have reported on the frequency of rotator cuff tearing in osteoarthritis, and this varies from 2%-11%.

The most significant operative variation to recognize and treat is posterior glenoid erosion with a tendency for posterior subluxation of the humerus. Treatment options include placing the glenoid in retrotilt, flattening the anterior aspect of the glenoid, or building up the posterior aspect of the glenoid. This latter method can be done by three techniques:

- building up the defect with cement, with or without screws
- using a bone graft
- using a special component.

All of these techniques have been utilized. At present it seems that bone grafting is the most acceptable alternative (Fig. 2). If the glenoid is allowed to remain in retrotilt, posterior instability will develop.

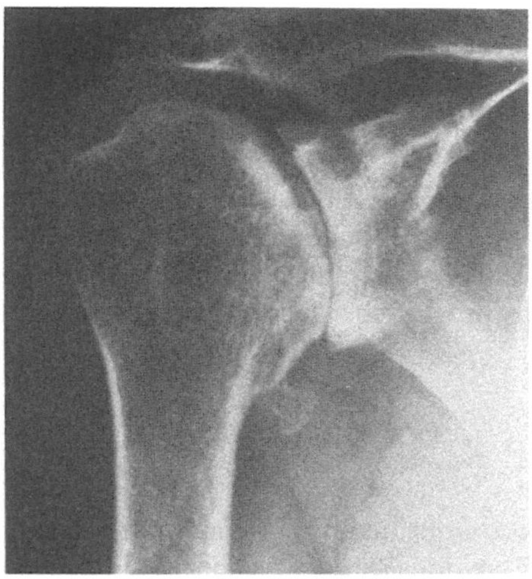

**Fig. 1.** Typical radiographic appearance of the osteoarthritic shoulder

Shoulder Replacement
Eds.: Kölbel/Helbig/Blauth

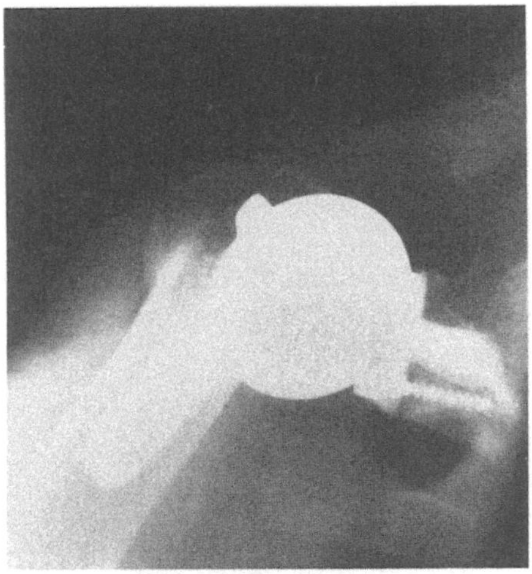

**Fig. 2.** Axillary radiograph of a patient with osteoarthritis following total shoulder replacement arthroplasty. Posterior glenoid erosion required bone grafting before insertion of the component. The graft is approximately 5 mm thick and is held in place with a screw

In our 31 patients with osteoarthritis, active abduction averaged 86° preoperatively and 141° postoperatively. Twenty-one of the 31 patients had more than 150° of active abduction [1].

## Rheumatoid Arthritis

There is great variability among patients with rheumatoid arthritis. Some of the problems associated with rheumatoid shoulder surgery were mentioned in an earlier presentation. These, of course, include glenoid loosening if the component is positioned in bone that is too osteoporotic, or if there is significant central glenoid erosion. Additionally, patients with severe rotator cuff involvement can have postoperative tearing of the rotator cuff repair.

Osteoporosis and the poor quality of fascial structures engender two intraoperative complications:

1) humeral shaft fracture and
2) traction injuries of the brachial plexus.

In our group of 29 patients, active abduction improved from 57° preoperatively to 102° postoperatively. Eighteen of the patients had abduction past 90°. When abduction was less than 90°, the patients either had severe rotator cuff involvement or were unable to participate actively in a therapy program because of their severe generalized rheumatoid disease.

## Old Trauma

Total shoulder replacement for old trauma is complicated by bone malposition and extensive scarring. This is particularly true if previous surgery has been performed. Another complicating feature is bone loss resulting from earlier surgical procedures. In our 13 patients with traumatic arthritis who underwent total shoulder arthroplasty, active abduction improved from 94° preoperatively to 109° postoperatively. In cases where 90° of active abduction was not obtained, a complication had occurred. Complications in this group included tuberosity nonunion, recurrent shoulder instability, rotator cuff tearing, and intraoperative nerve injury.

## Grading of Results

We graded our results after the system devised by Neer, categorizing patients as excellent, satisfactory, or unsatisfactory [2]. A separate group of patients was defined as having limited rehabilitation goals. These "limited goals" patients had major rotator cuff tearing that could be repaired only tenuously, and they participated in a different postoperative therapy program aimed at maintaining stability rather than regaining movement.

When graded by the Neer method, 20 of the 31 patients with osteoarthritis had excellent results, 2 satisfactory, and 7 unsatisfactory. In the 29 patients with rheumatoid arthritis, there were 5 excellent, 16 satisfactory, and 7 unsatisfactory results. The 13 patients with old trauma had 4 excellent, 6 satisfactory, and 3 unsatisfactory results. Of the osteoarthritics with unsatisfactory results, three had glenoid loosening necessitating revision surgery, one had glenoid loosening and pain, one had postoperative rotator cuff tearing with decreased motion, and one had reflex dystrophy. One patient also had unexplained pain. In the rheumatoid cases, all seven unsatisfactory results were attributed to failure to obtain 90° of active abduction. Of the traumatic arthritics with unsatisfactory results, one patient obtained only 80° of active abduction, and the other 3 had a complication that limited active motion. Three patients were classified as having limited rehabilitation goals. These goals were successfully accomplished in two.

## Cuff-Tear Arthropathy

Cuff-tear arthropathy has been recognized as a rare entity and was recently defined by Neer [3]. It includes a massive, longstanding rotator cuff tear associated with loss of glenohumeral cartilage and frequent distortion of the bony architecture. Usually the X-ray picture is very characteristic, but occasionally, when hypertrophic growth occurs, it may simulate osteoarthritis (Fig. 3).

From 1976 to 1982 we operated on 20 shoulders with cuff-tear arthropathy and performed some type of prosthetic replacement. Fourteen patients with 16 shoulders were alive and available for review at an average of 43 months. All had physical examination more than one year after surgery, and X-ray evaluation at more than two years. The patients consisted of 9 women and 5 men ranging in age from 53 to 79 years (average 68 years). Surgical treatment included rotator cuff repair in 12 shoulders, often using transposition techniques. A proximal humeral replacement was done in four shoulders, a standard Neer total shoulder arthroplasty in eight shoulders, and total shoulder replacement incorporating a hooded glenoid component in four shoulders.

Postoperatively pain was absent or mild in only 7 of the shoulders (44%). Pain relief was not clearly better with any particular treatment method, although when

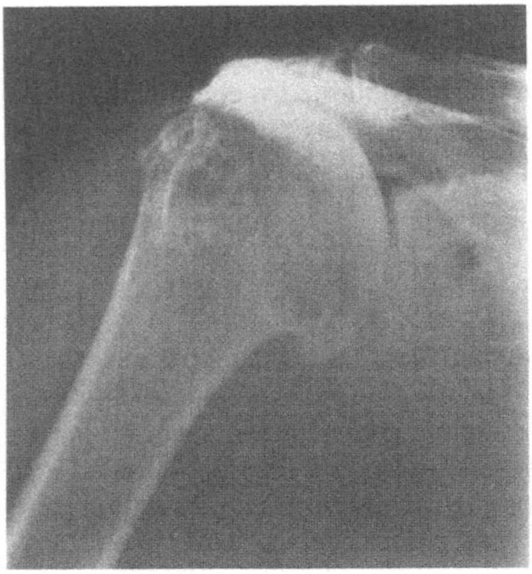

**Fig. 3.** Woman 73 years of age with long-standing rotator cuff tear who now manifests cartilage loss in the glenohumeral joint: cuff-tear arthropathy

pain relief was achieved, its quality seemed better with total arthroplasty than with proximal humeral replacement alone. Movement following surgery was not as good as with total arthroplasty in the three diagnostic groups defined above. Only 8 shoulders (50%) attained more than 90° of active abduction. It seemed quite clear in these patients that the hooded glenoid component offered no advantages in regaining active abduction over the other two methods with rotator cuff repair.

Six of the shoulders (38%) developed complications. These consisted of rotator cuff tearing in three, glenoid loosening in two, and dislocation in one patient with a hooded glenoid. Despite these difficulties, 12 of the 16 patients felt that they had benefitted from their surgery.

We concluded from this experience that cuff-tear arthropathy is very difficult to treat. There is no distinct advantage to a hooded glenoid component, and improved tendon repair techniques seem to be the best direction to pursue for better results in this treatment group.

## Summary

Relating prognosis to diagnosis, we may conclude that all diagnostic categories except cuff-tear arthropathy seem to experience excellent pain relief. The best motion and strength are achieved in *osteoarthritis*. Unfortunately, osteoarthritis also is associated with the highest loosening rate, and posterior glenoid erosion and instability are a constant concern.

In *rheumatoid arthritis* there is much variability because of the polyarticular involvement, rotator cuff changes, and capsular scarring.

In *traumatic arthritis* there is capsular and pericapsular scarring, especially if previous surgery has been performed. Bone loss may be a problem if bone was excised at earlier surgery. Tuberosity malunion certainly can occur.

*Cuff-tear arthropathy* is difficult to treat. It has the highest complication rate, and retearing of the rotator cuff is common. It appears that improved tendon repair techniques may offer the best hope for improving the prognosis in this difficult diagnostic category.

## References

1. Cofield RH (1984) Total shoulder arthroplasty with the Neer prosthesis. J Bone Joint Surg [Am] 66: 899-906
2. Neer CS II, Watson KC Stanton, FJ (1982) Recent experience in total shoulder replacement. J Bone Joint Surg [Am] 64: 319-337
3. Neer CS II, Craig EV, Fukuda H (1983) Cuff-tear arthropathy. J Bone Joint Surg [Am] 65: 1232-1244

## Discussion

*Blauth:* In presenting your results and the instances of loosening that occurred in the osteoarthritic group, you spoke of a particular group that was prone to that complication. What kinds of osteoarthritis were you referring to?

*Cofield:* I was referring to degenerative changes in general. As I tried to show, these patients have a fairly consistent pathology, and I did not single out a particular subgroup that would be distinguished from the rest by proneness to loosening.

*Lettin:* I have had little experience with primary osteoarthritis, apparently because we see it so infrequently. Can you tell us the prevalence of this disease among your patients? Also, it seems to me that the distinction you draw between osteoarthritis and cuff-tear arthropathy is really only a difference in the severity of degenerative changes. In my opinion, cuff-tear arthropathy is actually an osteoarthritis with associated secondary erosion of the rotator cuff. I would be interested to hear your views on this.

*Cofield:* About one-third of our patients who require shoulder replacement have osteoarthritis; the remaining two-thirds have rheumatoid arthritis and posttraumatic conditions with small subgroups.

What does cuff-tear arthropathy mean? Some of my colleagues consider it a variety of gouty arthritis in which crystalline deposits incite release of enzymes from synovial cells, which then destroy the cartilage and tendons. That is one hypothesis. But we also see patients who have extensive degenerative changes and cuff tears for years before developing osteoarthritis. In these cases it is obvious that the cuff tears came first, and that the osteoarthritis was secondary. I believe it is very significant that the rotator cuff is normal in osteoarthritics, and that massive defects exist in patients with cuff-tear arthropathy. Although both groups can have extensive damage to the joint surfaces, cuff-tear arthropathy is clearly distinct from osteoarthritis, and I do not believe that the difference between these entities is simply one of degree.

*Chairman:* Cuff-tear arthropathy with contact between the humeral head and acromion develops swiftly after traumatic dislocations and massive rotator cuff tears. Metaplastic new bone forms relatively quickly on the humeral head and acromion, and the glenohumeral joint surfaces degenerate very rapidly as a result of the subluxation. In these cases it is easy to trace the development of secondary changes following the cuff lesions. It is important to recognize the distinction between this condition and primary osteoarthritis of the shoulder. I feel strengthened in my caution about using prosthetic replacement for cuff-tear arthropathy. It would surely bring discredit on the Neer prosthesis if it were to be placed without also doing a meticulous repair of the rotator cuff and restoring the relation between the humerus and scapula.

# Shoulder Replacement for Bone Tumors

# Surgical Resection of Malignant Bone Tumors of the Shoulder Region - Indications and Results

K. Knahr, M. Salzer, M. Salzer-Kuntschik

When biopsy confirms the diagnosis of a *malignant bone tumor* after preliminary clinical and radiographic evaluation, and surgical resection is deemed necessary, it must be decided whether this can be accomplished only by amputating the affected limb, or whether a local resection can be done that would allow preservation of the limb.

Every *primary malignant bone tumor* must be radically removed according to the principles of oncologic surgery. This requires resection of the tumor with an adequate margin of healthy tissue, without opening the tumor capsule [7, 15]. A radical procedure of this kind is the only means for preventing a recurrence. A local recurrence signifies failure of the resective treatment and threatens the life of the patient.

Surgical resection may likewise be indicated for a *metastatic bone tumor*, especially if it is a "solitary" deposit from a renal or thyroid carcinoma. Again, a radical resection is needed just as for a primary neoplasm. When metastasis is more generalized, this procedure is unnecessary, and the main intent is to protect against painful pathologic fractures and hasten rehabilitation.

The type of surgical treatment indicated for malignant bone tumors of the proximal humerus depends on the diagnosis and especially on the extent of the tumor. The best techniques for assessing tumor extent in the bone are plain radiography and local bone scans. Tomography usually does not yield any additional information. The decision whether to amputate or perform a local resection depends chiefly on the amount of tumor spread to the soft tissues. This is most accurately assessed by angiography (see Fig. 2a) and computed tomography (see Fig. 1b).

First and foremost, the choice of surgical treatment must be dictated by oncologic requirements. Complete eradication of the tumor is the first priority. Under no circumstances should an inadequae resection be performed in the interest of preserving function. First the surgeon must establish the necessary extent of the resection according to oncologic criteria; only then may he consider ways of optimizing the functional result. Preservation of the hand is most important in this regard, for it cannot be adequately replaced by even the most sophisticated prosthesis. Hand salvage is advised even when two or three major nerves have to be sacrificed to ensure a radical removal, leaving only digital sensation and minimal residual function.

Based on these considerations, we have treated the majority of malignant bone tumors in recent years by local resection, reserving interscapulothoracic amputation and disarticulation at the shoulder joint for cases in which the entire neurovascular bundle is involved by tumor.

Shoulder Replacement
Eds.: Kölbel/Helbig/Blauth

## Amputation

### Interscapulothoracic (Forequarter) Amputation

This very radical operation is indicated when the malignancy has spread to involve the neurovascular bundle. In these cases it is impossible to preserve a functional upper limb and still get an adequate resection [4, 9, 17].

### Disarticulation at the Shoulder Joint

Amputation at this level is very rarely indicated for primary malignancies of the humerus [11] and is mainly reserved for tumors of the distal humerus. Disarticulation at the shoulder joint also may be the only treatment option for cases with extensive metastatic destruction.

## Resections

### Scapulectomy

Total scapulectomy is appropriate only for scapular malignancies located an adequate distance from the neurovascular bundle and glenohumeral joint [1, 2]. In many cases good hand and elbow function can be preserved by fixation of the humeral head to the chest wall (Fig. 1 a,c).

### Tikhor-Linberg Resection

This procedure involves an en bloc resection of the scapula, proximal humerus, and lateral part of the clavicle. It is indicated for malignant tumors of the proximal humerus or scapula that are close to the glenohumeral joint but do not yet involve the neurovascular bundle [8, 10]. This resection of the shoulder girdle is a mutilating procedure that results in complete loss of function of the shoulder joint. Nevertheless, it is reasonable to implant a prosthesis even in these cases, as this improves the function of the elbow (Fig. 2 b-d) and significantly extends the action radius of the hand.

Occasionally in the Tickhor-Linberg procedure it is necessary to include a portion of the chest wall in the resection to obtain an adequate surgical margin.

### Resection of the Proximal Humerus

Resection of the proximal humerus alone can provide radical control of bone malignancy only if there is little or no soft-tissue involvement, so that the neurovascular bundle can be preserved without compromising oncologic demands. Occasionally the resection must include the radial nerve because of its proximity to the bone. These cases will still have reasonable residual function of the forearm and hand, and so division of the radial nerve is not a contraindication to resective treatment. By bridging the defect with a prosthesis, one can markedly improve the function of the elbow and thus the overall function of the arm (Fig. 3 a,b) [3, 4].

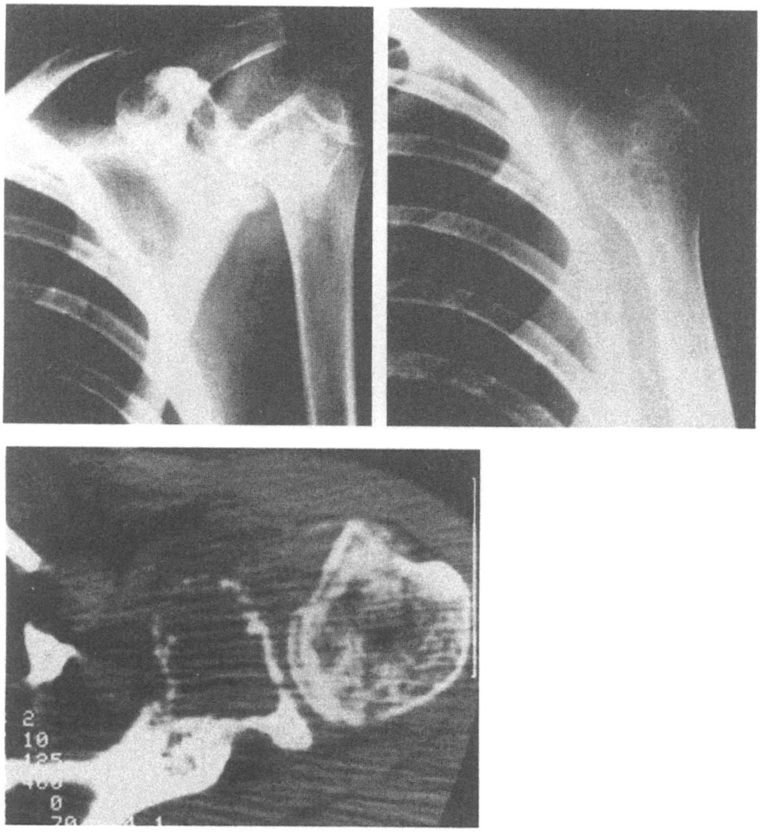


a c

b

**Fig. 1a-c.** S. W., male, 26 years, Ewing's sarcoma of left scapula. **a** Preoperative plain radiograph yields no information on tumor size. **b** CT clearly demonstrates the large soft-tissue mass. **c** Follow-up radiograph 16 months after total scapulectomy

### Total Resection of the Humerus

With an intraosseous tumor that extends far distally, the humerus must be disarticulated at the elbow and removed in toto. Bracing of the arm provides a definitive treatment and enables good hand function through the passive position change (Fig. 4a,b). It remains to be seen whether the few cases treated with a prosthetic implant will have equally good elbow function in the long term [6].

## Technique of Proximal Humeral Resection with Insertion of a Prosthesis

The operating technique depends on the extent of the tumor. Thus, we are unable to present a step-by-step technique, since one always must be guided by individual requirements. Nevertheless, some general principles can be stated:

The skin incision should circumvent all biopsy scars so that those areas can be included in the resection. Usually the incision is made in the deltopectoral groove. The neurovascular bundle is identified distal to the tumor and is carefully isolated a

b

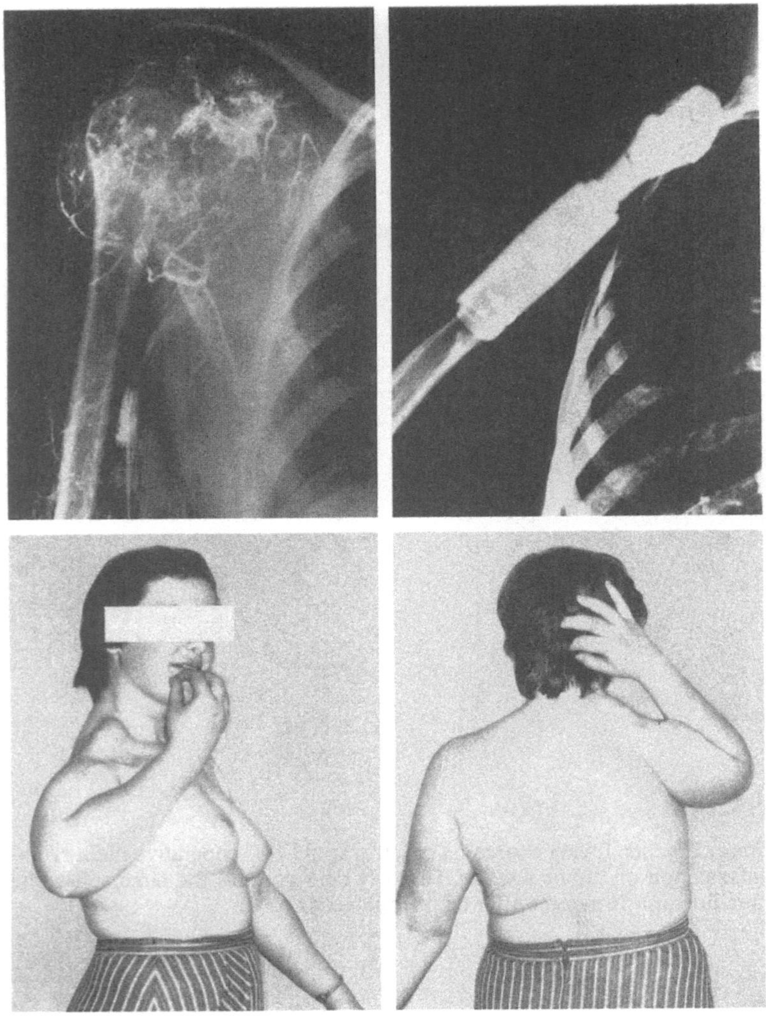

c

d

**Fig. 2 a-d.** E. R., female, 16 years, fibrosarcoma of right shoulder. **a** Angiographic appearance of the extensive soft-tissue tumor. **b** Follow-up radiograph 9 years after Tikhor-Linberg resection and insertion of a ceramic prosthesis. **c,d** Functional result is very good; patient is self-sufficient with everyday tasks

from the tumor into the axillary region. The pectoralis major muscle is divided at its insertion, as are the teres minor, latissimus dorsi, and subscapularis coursing from the chest wall to the humerus. The muscles arising from the coracoid (short biceps, coracobrachialis) can occasionally be preserved. Many times it is necessary to divide the axillary nerve. All muscles in direct apposition to the tumor are included in the resection. This may involve different portions of the deltoid, brachialis, biceps, and triceps muscles, depending on the location of the tumor. While it would be favorable in terms of prosthetic attachment to preserve portions of the rotator cuff and joint capsule, a radical operation usually necessitates the removal of these structures.

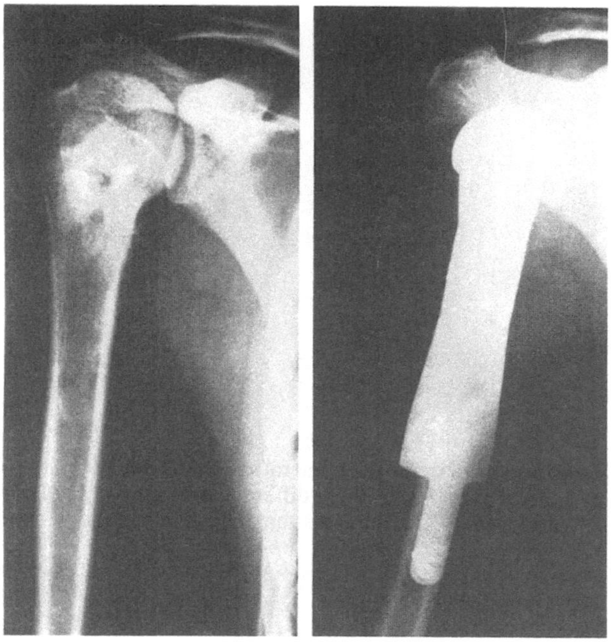

a b

**Fig. 3a,b.** H. C., male, 18 years, metastatic osteosarcoma of the right proximal humerus. **a** Predominantly intraosseous destruction of the proximal humerus. **b** Follow-up radiograph 42 months after insertion of a metallic tumor prosthesis

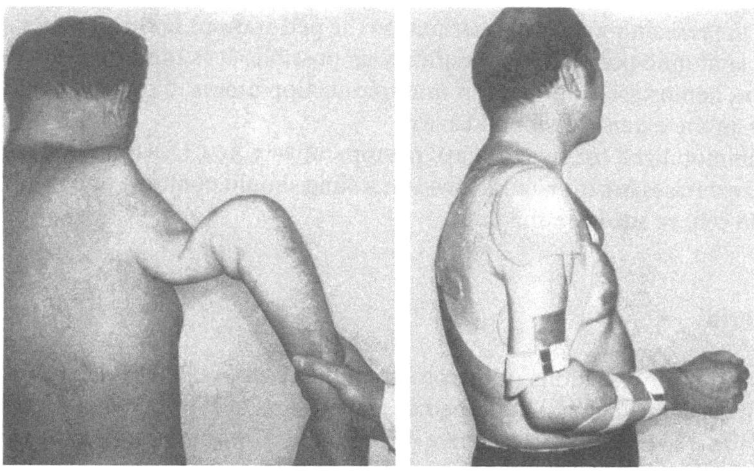

a b

**Fig. 4a,b.** E. A., male, 39 years, fibrosarcoma of right humerus. **a** Status after tumor resection without prosthetic replacement. **b** Appearance after insertion of a shoulder prosthesis with a locking elbow joint

Following the en bloc removal of the tumor, we reshape the humeral stump with a conical cutting tool and press-fit the prosthesis onto the tapered stump (Fig. 5 a). While we use a screw to secure ceramic implants against rotation, the metal prostheses are equipped with straps that give rotational stability and also provide a certain tension-band effect (Fig. 5 c).

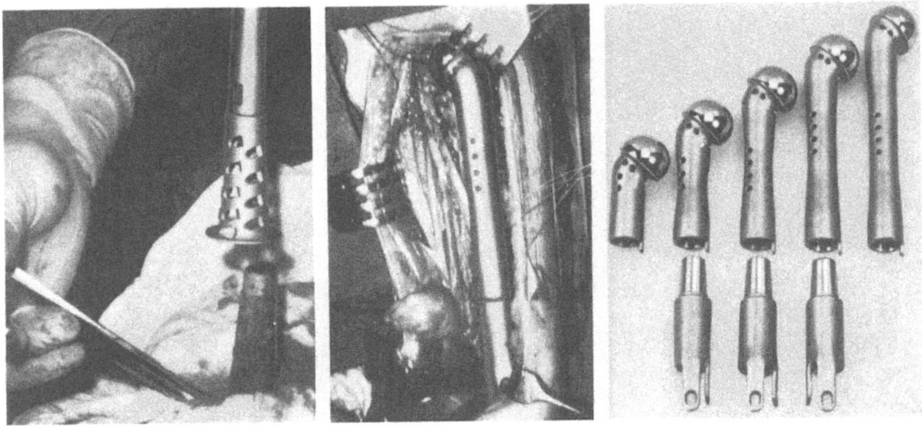

a b c

**Fig. 5. a** A special conical cutting tool is used to shape the humeral stump. **b** Operative site after placement of the prosthesis. **c** Modular system with three different cone sizes (17-21 mm diameters) and 5 spacers (100-220 mm lengths). The humerus-femur system includes a cone with a 24-mm diameter

The length of the implant should be such that the head of the prosthesis is positioned just beneath the humeral vault; it is set in about 15°-20° of retrotorsion (Fig. 5b). Reconstruction of the muscles depends on the amount of musculature that remains. The goal is to achieve maximum muscular coverage of the implant and to reattach the remaining muscle insertions to the perforations in the prosthesis, matching their anatomic positions as accurately as possible. It is important to obtain a meticulous hemostasis and to insert multiple suction drains to prevent hematoma formation in the extensive wound cavity.

The limb is immobilized for several days postoperatively in a Desault bandage, and then gentle exercises are initiated. However, a sling should continue to be worn for some time to relieve stress on the joint.

## Clinical Material

We performed 42 tumor resections of the proximal humerus and subsequent prosthetic replacements at the General Orthopedics Department of Wien-Gersthof Hospital from 1974 to 1984. The patients were 15 men and 27 women ranging in age from 8 to 74 years (average 32.8 years). The underlying disease was osteosarcoma in 13 patients, chondrosarcoma in 7 patients, Ewing's sarcoma in 3, malignant lymphoma in 2, and 1 case each of plasmocytoma, fibrosarcoma, and malignant fibrous histiocytoma. Eleven patients had metastatic bone tumors. In three patients with primary bone tumors that had been previously treated elsewhere by local radiation or chemotherapy, we were unable to make a definitive diagnosis from the surgical specimen.

## Oncologic Results

The surgical margins in our population were assessed using the Surgical Staging System of Enneking et al. (1980). All 13 osteosarcomas were classified as Stage IIB. Of the 7 chondrosarcomas, 1 was a low-grade malignancy (Stage IB), and the remaining 6 were high-grade (Stage IIB). Because this classification excludes hematologic and metastatic tumors, we limited our analysis of surgical margins to the osteosarcomas and chondrosarcomas.

It is imperative that every malignant tumor be excised with a surrounding cuff of normal tissue. This requires at least a "wide" surgical margin according to the Staging System of Enneking et al. We obtained a wide margin in only 2 osteosarcomas and 4 chondrosarcomas, while the remaining 11 osteosarcomas and 3 chondrosarcomas were classified as "marginal" (resection performed through reactive tissue around the lesion).

Clinical follow-up indicates that of the 11 marginally resected osteosarcoma patients, 7 are alive and free of disease after 18-131 months (average 58.1 months), while 4 died after 6-18 months. One of the patients who died also had a local recurrence. All 3 of the chondrosarcoma patients with marginal resections are alive after a follow-up of 42-92 months.

Of the 2 "widely" resected osteosarcoma patients, 1 is alive after a relatively short follow-up interval of 8 months, and the other died from generalized metastasis after 15 months. Of the 4 chondrosarcoma patients with wide resections, 2 are alive after follow-ups of 16 and 46 months, and the other 2 died after 11 and 29 months.

When we evaluate the humeral resection in terms of its oncologic efficacy, we unfortunately find that the surgical procedure was insufficient in nearly three-fourths of the osteosarcoma and chondrosarcoma patients according to the criteria of Enneking et al. The major problem is the soft-tissue component of the tumor. With all 11 marginally resected osteosarcomas, "wide" margins were obtained as far as the bony resection was concerned, but the resection was "marginal" in terms of the soft tissues. Even so, the clinical results in our series are not as bad as one would expect from the inadequate surgical margins. The survival rate of the 11 marginally resected osteosarcoma patients (all with pre- and postoperative high-dosage methotrexate therapy) is 63.6% with an average follow-up of 58.1 months and is comparable to the results of surgical treatment in the COSS-80 study [20]. Even so, these results cannot be regarded as satisfactory.

The protocol of New York Memorial Hospital must be recommended for osteosarcomas of the proximal humerus: After preoperative chemotherapy, all patients undergo a Tikhor-Linberg resection of the shoulder girdle. This is followed by high-dosage combination chemotherapy. The results of this approach are impressive: no local recurrences, and 23 of 25 patients (92%) are alive and free of disease after an average of 5 years [13].

## Prosthesis

The *ceramic prosthesis* is a modular device that was formerly manufactured by the Rosenthal company [14]. It consists of a conical anchoring element, spacer, and head. The modular design allows to assemble the implant individually according to the extent of the resection. It is inserted without cement. After the manufacturer discontinued production of this implant, a *metallic modular prosthesis* was developed in cooperation with Aesculap Instruments which incorporates the same design principle (see Fig. 5 c). Tension-band straps were attached to the cone to improve the stability of the anchorage and check rotational displacement [16, 19]. A major advantage of the conical sleeve attachment over conventional stem anchorage [3, 5, 12, 18] is that it permits stable fixation of the prosthesis to the humeral stump even after extensive resections.

## Complications (Table 1)

### Implant Loosening

Twenty-four ceramic and 18 metallic implants were placed in the 42 patients who underwent proximal humeral resections. Twenty of the ceramic prosthesis are still stable after follow-ups of 3-131 months (average 49.2 months). In 4 of the ceramic prostheses, loosening at the bone-cone interface occurred between 12 and 80 months postoperatively. In one case the loosening was caused by trauma and in two others by local infection. One woman has no complaints despite the loosening and so has not consented to reoperation.

### Infections

Four cases of early infection were observed. In one case the prosthesis was removed without revision at 3 weeks postoperatively and in another case at 12 months. Two patients died at 5 and 12 months from their underlying disease. No reoperations were required.

### Other Complications

One patients manifested delayed healing postoperatively, but that resolved with conservative care. The number of subluxations and dislocations is relatively high, affecting a total of eight patients. This high incidence is due to the lack of soft-tissue coverage of the implant occasioned by the extensive tumor resection. The functional effects of the subluxations and dislocations are mild, however.

**Table 1.** Complications Following Prosthetic Replacement of the Proximal Humerus (n = 42)

| | Stable | Major complications | | Minor complications (subluxation, delayed wound healing) |
|---|---|---|---|---|
| | | Loosening | Infection | |
| Ceramic implant (n = 24) | 20 | 4 (12-80 months) | 4 (1-2 weeks) | 8 |
| Metallic implant (n = 18) | 17 | 1 (30 months) | 0 | 3 |
| Total | 37 | 5 | 4 | 11 |

## Conclusions

The local resection of malignant bone tumors of the shoulder joint presents a great challenge to the orthopedist who deals with cancer patients. Oncologic requirements and the need to preserve a serviceable hand are the two crucial factors which determine the choice of a surgical procedure. Always, of course, the preservation of life (= adequate surgical margins) takes precedence over functional considerations.

Analysis of our own material has shown that with osteosarcoma, the most common primary malignant bone tumor of the proximal humerus, we were unable to achieve a "wide" (adequate) resection in 11 of the 13 tumors treated. For this reason a Tikhor-Linberg resection should be mandatory for all osteosarcomas of the proximal humerus. By inserting a prosthesis and attaching its head to the chest wall, it is possible to achieve a functional outcome that is almost as satisfying as after resection of the humerus alone.

The uncemented conical anchorage has proved effective in the tumor prosthesis developed by us. Its advantage over prostheses with anchoring stems is that it enables prosthetic replacement even when the humerus has been resected at a very low level. Modular components were developed to avoid the need for time-consuming custom fabrication. This ensures that an appropriate prosthesis will always be available for each patient.

## References


1. Bacci G, Campanacci M, Pagani A (1978) Adjuvant chemotherapy in the treatment of clinically localised Ewing's sarcoma. J Bone Joint Surg [Br] 60: 567-574
2. Becker F, Becker W (1968) Operative Behandlung der Tumoren der Knochen, der Gelenke und Weichteile des Stützgewebes. In: Holder E, Meythaler F, du Mesnil de Rochemont R (Hrsg) Therapie maligner Tumoren, Hämoblastome und Hämoblastosen, Bd II. Encke, Stuttgart, S 791
3. Burri C, Rüter A (1977) Prothesen und Alternativen am Arm, Teil I: Schultergelenk. Huber, Bern
4. Campanacci M, Laus M (1980) Local recurrence after amputation for osteosarcoma. J Bone Joint Surg [Br] 62: 201-207
5. Campanacci M, Calderoni P, Cervellati C, Guerra A, Calderoni P (1983) Modular rotatory endoprosthesis for segmental resection of the proximal humerus. In: Chao EYS, Ivins JC (eds) Tumor prostheses for bone and joint reconstruction. Thieme-Stratton, New York
6. Engelbrecht E, Siegel A, Röttger J, Heinert K (1980) Erfahrungen mit der Anwendung von Schultergelenksprothesen. Chirurg 51: 794-800
7. Enneking WF, Spanier SS, Goodman MA (1980) A system for surgical staging of musculoskeletal sarcoma. Clin Orthop 153: 106-120
8. Kotz R, Salzer M (1975) Resection therapy of malignant tumors of the shoulder girdle. Oesterr Z Onkol 2: 97
9. Marcove RC, Mike V, Hajek JV, Levin AG, Hutter RVP (1970) Osteogenic sarcoma under the age of twenty-one. A review of onehundred and forty-five operative cases. J Bone Joint Surg [Am] 52: 411-423
10. Marcove RC, Lewis MM, Huvos AG (1977) En-bloc upper humeral interscapulo-thoracic resektion. Clin Orthop 124: 219-228
11. Mc Kenna RJ, Schwinn CP, Soong KY, Higinbotham NL (1966) Sarcomata of the osteogenic series, osteosarcoma, fibrosarcoma, chondrosarcoma, parosteal osteogenic sarcoma and sarcoma arising in abnormal bone. J Bone Joint Surg [Am] 48: 1-26
12. Neer II ChS (1983) Design and technical considerations for proximal humerus and shoulder prostheses. In: Chao EYS, Ivins JC (eds) Tumor prostheses for bone and joint reconstruction. Thieme-Stratton, New York

13. Rosen G (1985) Preoperative (neoadjuvant) chemotherapy for osteogenic sarcoma: A ten year experience. Orthopedics vol 8/5: 659-664
14. Salzer M, Knahr K, Locke H, Stärk N, Matejowsky Z, Plenk H jr, Punzei G, Zweymüller K (1979) A bioceramic endoprosthesis for the replacement of the proximal humerus. Arch Orthop Trauma Surg 93: 169-184
15. Salzer M, Knahr K, Salzer-Kuntschik M (1977) Indications for radical resection of malignant bone tumours. Results in forty-six cases. Ital J Orthop Traumatol 3: 155-166
16. Salzer M, Knahr K (1983) Design problems - cement-free anchorage of tumor prostheses. In: Chao EYS, Ivins JC (eds) Tumor prostheses for bone and joint reconstruction. Thieme-Stratton, New York
17. Sim FH, Pritchard DJ, Ivins JC (1977) Forequarter amputation. Orthop Clin North 8/4: 921-931
18. Sim FH, Pritchard DJ, Chao EYS (1983) Prosthetic replacement of the proximal humerus. In: Chao EYS, Ivins IC (eds) Tumor prostheses for bone and joint reconstruction. Thieme-Stratton, New York
19. Ungethüm M, Knahr K, Salzer M, Blömer W (1983) Zementfrei zu implantierende Spezialprothesen nach dem Baukastenprinzip für den proximalen Femur - und Humeruser-satz. Med Orthop Tech 4: 104-113
20. Winkler K, Beron G, Kotz R et al. (1985) Einfluß des lokalchirurgischen Vorgehens auf die Inzidenz von Metastasen nach neoadjuvanter Chemotherapie des Osteosarkoms. Z Orthop (in press)

## Discussion

*Chairman:* How much do the components of your modular system weigh?

*Knahr:* The system is made of titanium and is relatively lightweight. The prostheses are lighter than ceramic prostheses.

*Chairman:* Bone cement usually is a factor in loosening when it is used to compensate for deficiencies in the insertion and orientation of an implant. It will correct for these deficiencies for a certain period of time, but ultimately the system will fail. I believe that cement fixation has excellent longevity when it is used properly, i.e., as recommended by Charnley, and that bone cement should not be discredited equally for all applications.

*Knahr:* At our center we are very skeptical about bone cement. We have not had major problems in the proximal humerus. But with tumor prostheses about the knee joint, where stresses are much greater, we have had definite loosening problems with bone cement.

*Chairman:* The bone sees only the surface of the implant and reacts to the load imposed by that surface. Regardless of whether it is bone cement or metal: if it is done well, it will hold; if it is done poorly, it will not.

*Blauth:* I am surprised by the stability figure of 88% that you obtained with the conical attachment. I have reservations that this type of anchorage will really do what you expect in the long term. Are there problems with the viability of the bone stump on which the cone is placed, and do critical zones exist in the humerus with regard to blood flow? Where are they located, what kinds of experience have you had, and how long have you been following these cases?

*Knahr:* With the ceramic prostheses we have a minimum of 5 years' follow-up and a maximum of 9 years. We no longer used ceramic prostheses after that time, because the manufacturer stopped making them. Twenty of 24 prostheses have remained stable. With the metallic prostheses, we presently have follow-ups from 1 to 5 years. The 88% figure pertains to the total number.

We have seen instances of prosthetic loosening in our patients. In these cases we immobilized the limb for a certain period of time, during which the devices completely restabilized and consolidated.

Time and again in our patients with metastases we note continued viability of the humeral stump. Presumably the conical attachment works in the upper arm because of the relatively low mechanical stresses in that area. We have also tried the conical attachment in tumor prostheses for the knee, but all of them failed; the same is true of the femur, at least in its distal portion. In the humerus, evidence to date indicates that the design is effective, although longer-term results are still needed.

# Functional Results after Prosthetic Replacement of the Proximal Humerus

J. Sekera and M. Salzer

Several surgical options exist for treating cases of malignant destruction of the proximal humerus:

1. Amputation - either disarticulation at the shoulder joint or interscapulothoracic amputation [1, 4, 5, 6, 9]
2. Resection without replacement [2, 3]
3. Resection followed by prosthetic replacement [7, 8]

In the last case we have used hemiarthroplasty exclusively. Our intent is to obtain a more serviceable upper extremity and especially to improve the function of the elbow joint, forearm, and hand.

To determine the functional status of an arm following this type of surgery, we reexamined our patients using the analysis sheet developed by Enneking. Because we felt that this evaluation did not yield sufficient information, we tried to extend the scope of the questions. We wished to assess the ability of the patient to be reintegrated into his social and working environment on the basis of his ability to perform normal daily activities.

## Clinical Material

From 1974 to 1984 we performed reconstructive hemiarthroplasties in 42 patients who underwent resections of malignant bone tumors of the proximal humerus at the Wien-Gersthof Orthopedic Hospital. The lesions were primary in 31 patients and metastatic in 12. Sixteen patients died from their disease before the start of follow-up. Eight patients from other countries were unavailable for follow-up, and two patients were followed for less than one year. Thus, a total of 16 patients were available for the present review. They consisted of 10 males and 6 females with an average age of 29 years (11-71 years). The average follow-up period was 62 months (14-132 months).

Four of the patients had chondrosarcoma, four had Ewing's sarcoma, three had osteosarcoma, and there was one case each of malignant fibrous histiocytoma and fibrosarcoma. Three patients had metastatic disease from 1) an osteosarcoma of the femur, 2) Ewing's sarcoma of the rib, and 3) thyroid carcinoma.

Seven of the patients were treated with a ceramic prosthesis, and nine with a metallic prosthesis. All of the replacements were hemiarthroplasties performed without cement [8]. The resection was done in the proximal third of the humerus in three patients, the middle third in eight patients, and the distal third in five.

All of the patients who presented for follow-up were free of local recurrence.

Shoulder Replacement
Eds.: Kölbel/Helbig/Blauth

## Complications

When we examined the articular relations of the operated shoulders, we found that the head of the prosthesis was centered in 10 patients; in 1 of these the head had been fixed to a rib after prior scapular resection. Dislocation was noted in four patients, and two others showed a clinically insignificant tendency toward subluxation.

At the time of the follow-up examination, the bony attachment of the prosthesis was clinically and radiographically solid in 14 of the 16 patients, and axial alignment was correct in all but 2 cases, which showed minor deviations.

Marked loosening was noted in 2 patients at 30 and 80 months postoperatively. However, both patients are doing well despite the loosening and do not desire reoperation at the present time.

One patient sustained a traumatic fracture of the prosthesis-bone attachment 54 months after implantation. The ceramic prosthesis was removed, and a metallic prosthesis was inserted. The follow-up period since reoperation is 43 months.

## Results

Six of the patients operated had less than 10° of active abduction. Seven patients could abduct their arm to 40°, and 3 could abduct it past 40°. Eleven of the 16 patients had less than 40° of forward flexion and more than 50° of external rotation, and 14 of the 16 patients had active internal rotation exceeding 60°.

Nine of the 16 patients were free of pain, and 2 reported intermittent pain. Three patients complained of pain on exertion, and two complained of constant pain.

## Enneking Evaluation

The analysis sheet devised by Enneking basically covers the following parameters:
- range of motion, joint status
- strength
- pain
- subjective attitude toward surgical outcome
- complications

Two of our 16 patients rated excellent according to this scheme, 6 good, 4 fair, and 4 poor.

Our *additional questions* assessed the ability of the patient to perform essential daily activities to determine his level of self-sufficiency versus reliance on outside help.

Twelve of the 16 patients had no problems with anal hygiene. Ten patients could cut their food themselves and raise it to their mouth with the operated hand. Fourteen patients had no problems with dressing or with personal hygiene.

Fourteen patients were able to sleep on the operated side without discomfort. Only four patients were able to comb their hair with the operated hand. Twelve of the 16 patients could carry objects weighing 5-10 kg.

When subjective attitudes were elicited, 3 of the 16 patients reported significant disability. Eight patients considered themselves mildly handicapped, and five patients felt that they had no handicap whatsoever.

While 6 of the 16 patients were only partially satisfied with the result of their operation, 10 patients were completely satisfied. None of the patients expressed dissatisfaction with the result.

When asked to name the most serious functional deficits of the operated arm, the patients gave varying responses, although certain trends are apparent. Patients were most frequently troubled by the inability to perform activities above their head. This was particularly true of younger patients who participated in sports activities. An entirely unexpected complaint, voiced by several patients, was the inability to raise the hand in a normal gesture of greeting. Apparently the lack of this gesture conveys a feeling of discrimination and reinforces their handicapped status.

On the positive side, the patients pronounced themselves able to perform a great variety of everyday activities including housework, occupational duties, handicrafts, eating, personal hygiene, and even athletic activities such as swimming, bicycling, tennis, and skiing. All the patients used certain "tricks" to accomplish these activities.

When we consider the extent of the humeral resection, we find that all the patients with proximal-third resections rated excellent to good. Four patients with middle-third resections rated excellent to good, and four rated fair to poor. As for the distal-third resections, only one of the five patients rated excellent to good, and the other four rated fair to poor.

## Summary

The limitation of function in the operated shoulder significantly limits the action radius of the hand. The less active function there is in the new shoulder joint, the less the value of the operated hand. However, the patients learn tricks to compensate for their deficiencies and do well despite their handicap.

Analysis reveals that patients who had less extensive resections fared better after surgery than patients who had greater lengths of the humerus resected.

In some patients we find a marked discrepancy between the objective assessment of arm function and the feeling of being handicapped. This is illustrated by the case of a 26-year-old woman with a pronounced dislocation of the prosthetic head, an associated flexion contracture of the elbow, and an extension loss of 60° after undergoing radiation therapy elsewhere. Despite these problems, the patient does not feel handicapped in any way and is satisfied with the result of her surgery.

On the other hand, a 21-year-old man who has 60° of active abduction, 90° of active forward flexion, and unrestricted rotation feels handicapped 43 months after his operation because he is unable to participate fully in certain types of sport.

Based on this experience, we have concluded that the extent of rehabilitation is certainly important but not necessarily crucial. A major factor is the ability of the patient to adjust to the situation as a whole. The question is whether he can deal with his natural fears and whether he has learned to accept his disabled arm, even if it cannot function normally in many areas. If he is able to do these things, and pain is not a problem, it will not matter how much motion he possesses or how much stress he can place on his operated arm.

By contrast, patients who do not become integrated into their environment will suffer from their disability and will be impaired by the defect which they feel condemns them to an inferior existence.

## References


1. El-Domeiri A, Miller T (1969) The role of interscapulothoracic amputation in the treatment of malignant tumors. Surg Gynecol Obstet 129: 1203-1206
2. Enneking WF (1983) Functional evaluation of reconstruction after tumor resection. 2nd International Workshop on the Design and Application of Tumor Prosthesis for Bone and Joint Reconstruction. Vienna, Sept 5-8, 1983
3. Kotz R, Salzer M (1975) Resection therapy of malignant tumours of the shoulder girdle. Österr Z Onkol 2/4: 97
4. Kotz R, Salzer M (1975) Erfahrung mit der Schulterresektion bei malignen Tumoren. Orthop Praxis 6: 427-431
5. Linberg BE (1928) Interscapulothoracic resection for malignant tumors of the shoulder joint region. J Bone Joint Surg 10: 344-349
6. Marcove RC, Lewis MM, Huvos AG (1977) En-bloc upper humeral interscapulo-thoracic resection. Clin Orthop 124: 219-228
7. Marcove RC, Rosen G (1980) En-bloc resections for osteogenic sarcoma. Cancer 45: 3040-3044
8. Salzer M, Knahr K (1983) Design problems - cementfree anchorage of tumor prostheses. In: Chao EYS, Ivins JC. Tumor prostheses for bone and joint reconstruction. Thieme-Stratton, New York, pp 361-365
9. Salzer M, Knahr K, Locker H, Stärk N, Matejowsky Z, Plenk H jr, Punzet G, Zweymüller K (1979) A bioceramic endoprosthesis for the replacement of the proximal humerus. Arch Orthop Trauma Surg 93: 169-184
10. Sim FH, Pritchard DJ, Ivins JC (1977) Forequarter amputation. Orthop Clin North Am 8/4: 921-931

# Tumor Prosthesis for the Shoulder

C. Burri

We are indebted to Albee [1] for introducing the surgical replacement of the resected proximal humerus. He used the head and proximal portion of the fibula for this purpose, but his results were not convincing. In the early 1950s, surgeons mainly in the U.S. began to use prostheses for replacement of the upper humerus. Venable [6], for example, described in 1952 a Vitallium prosthesis that was anchored in the humerus by means of a stem combined with a sheath and screws. R. Mathys [4] introduced a new type of shoulder tumor prosthesis made of plastic (polyacetal resin). We have used this type since 1972 because it offers significant advantages over metallic prostheses - most notably the ability to reattach osteotomized tendon insertions to the prosthesis with screws.

The proximal humerus is a site of predilection for tumors of bone. Benign tumors that have not damaged the joint surface and are amenable to surgical treatment should be curetted out and the defect filled with grafted bone. We feel that semimalignant tumors or tumors of low-grade malignancy are good indications for the insertion of a shoulder prosthesis. The same applies to solitary metastases, especially when associated with pathologic fractures. With malignant tumors, the prosthesis can provide an alternative to disarticulation as long as the process has not invaded the surrounding soft-tissues. If metastases from the malignancy are confirmed, precluding the possibility of amputation with life-saving intent, prosthetic treatment to preserve the arm may still be the best therapeutic option.

## Operative Technique

Generally the operation is done with the patient supine and the arm draped free for mobility. The skin incision starts proximally over the lateral border of the acromion, follows the anterior margin of the deltoid, and extends distally according to the necessary level of the resection through the humerus. The humeral shaft is exposed in the deltopectoral groove, lateral to the cephalic vein, by retraction of the overlying muscles. If the tumor extent permits limiting the resection to the proximal portion of the humerus, care should be taken to preserve the tendinous insertions so that an optimum functional result can be obtained. In more extensive tumor cases where disarticulation and interscapulothoracic amputation are not acceptable, it is necessary that radical surgical margins be obtained, i.e., that involved compartments be included in the resection [5]. From the outset it should be recognized that complete functional recovery is not a realistic goal, although the radial nerve and axillary nerve should be spared if at all possible.

Following the tumor resection, reaming of the humeral shaft is performed with the ASIF intramedullary instrument, and the bone end is reamed open in conical fashion to improve the seating of the prosthesis. The prosthesis (whose exact shank length can be determined only after radical resection of the tumor) is inserted by

Shoulder Replacement
Eds.: Kölbel/Helbig/Blauth

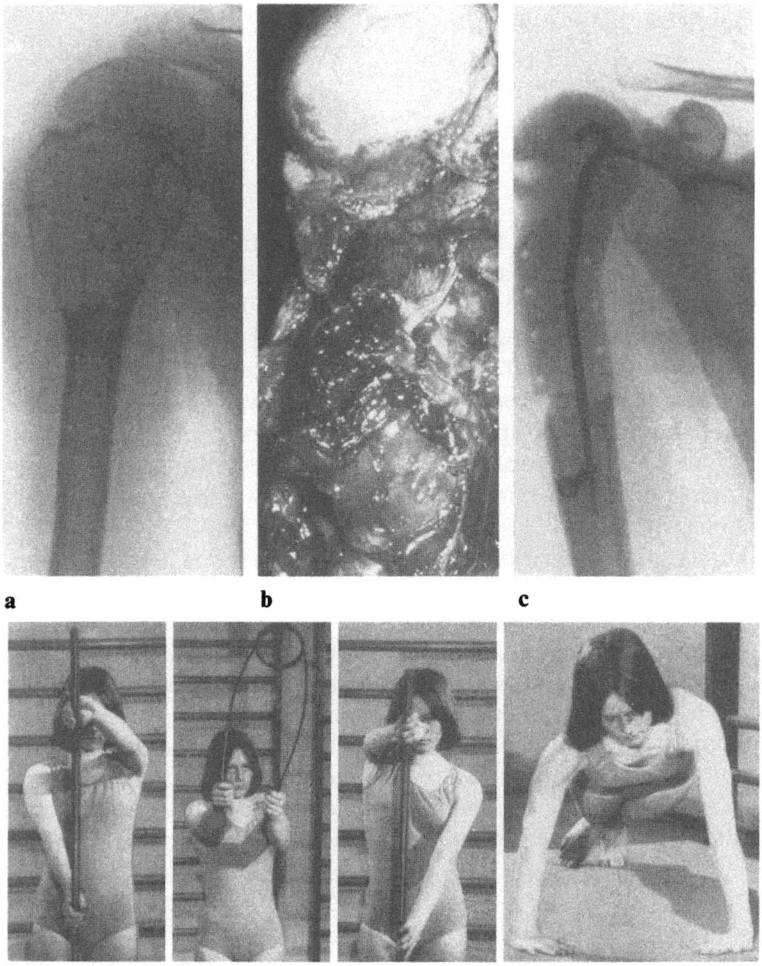

a b c

d

**Fig. 1 a-d.** Ten-year-old girl with grade II-III giant-cell tumor. **a** Preoperative radiograph. **b** Specimen - the tumor has transgressed the bone-periosteum boundary. **c** Postoperative radiograph. **d** Functional result more than 10 years after the operation

driving the stem into the medullary cavity of the residual humeral shaft in 10°-20° of increased retroversion. The stem is additionally secured with a small cortex screw inserted perpendicular to the shaft (Fig. 1 a-d).

Placement of the prosthesis is followed by a meticulous reconstruction of the soft tissues with reattachment of the tendinous insertions. If it was possible to release the insertions on small pieces of bone, these are attached to the prosthesis with screws, making sure that some type of bony continuity is established between the fragments and the residual humeral shaft. This can be done by packing autologous or homologous bone around the prosthetic stem. If the tumor resection precludes a bony reattachment of the tendons, we pass the long biceps tendon through the holes in the head of the prosthesis to form a kind of tendinous sheet, and we then tack the rotators onto that sheet. This technique has proved successful in our hands. We should emphasize that it is biologically impossible to suture soft tissues directly to plastic or

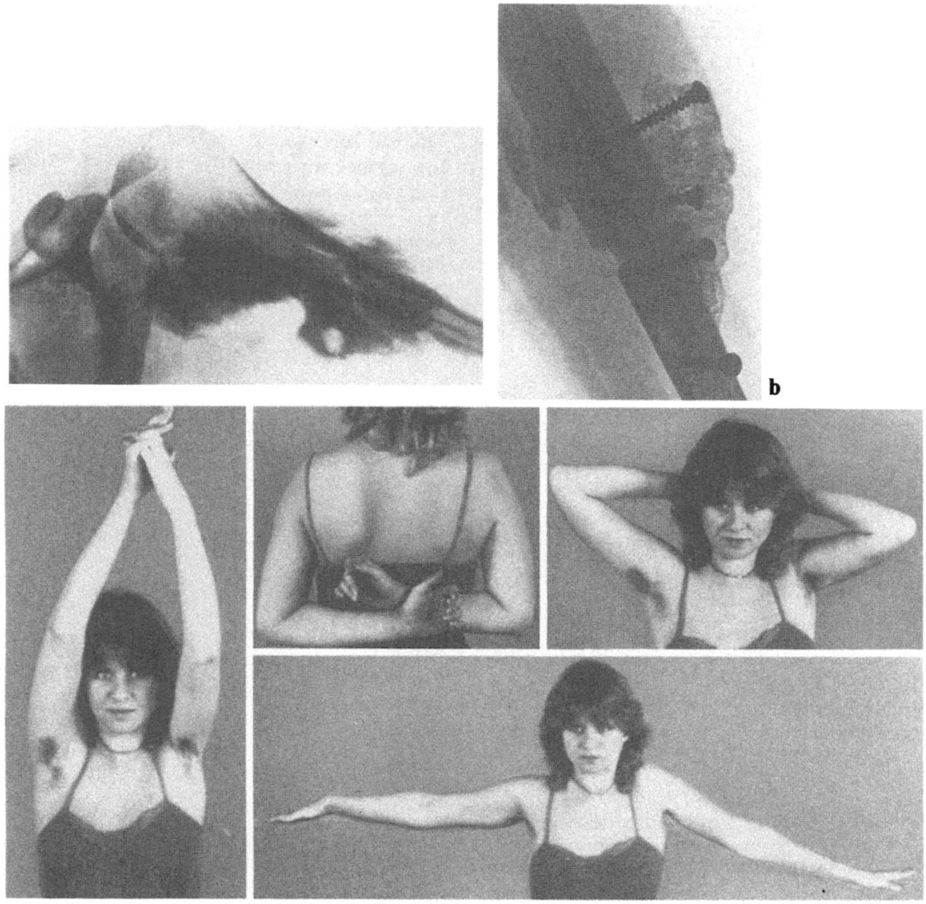

Fig. 2 a-c. Woman 22 years of age with parosteal sarcoma. a Preoperative radiograph. b Postoperative radiograph: The deltoid insertion has been reattached to the humerus on a corticocancellous graft. c Functional result

metal, and it is necessary to use alternative means as just described (Fig. 2 a-c). Two or three suction drains are placed at the conclusion of the operation, and the wound is closed in layers. Postoperatively the limb is placed on an abduction splint, and an effort is made to start assisted exercises from the splint. Active exercises may be done if the surgeon has achieved a stable, osseous reattachment of the muscular insertions. With a tendinous attachment, it is best to immobilize the limb on the abduction splint for several weeks.

## Results

We published results of shoulder tumor prostheses in a prior collective study [2, 3]. Since then we have been able to document a series of 68 patients, 58 of whom were available for follow-up. The tumors were primary in 25 patients and metastatic in 43. The most common primaries were chondrosarcomas (7), osteosarcomas (6), and

**Table 1.** Shoulder Tumor Prostheses (n = 68)

| Primary tumors | |
|---|---|
| Chondrosarcoma | 7 |
| Osteosarcoma | 6 |
| Giant-cell tumor | 8 |
| Spindle-cell sarcoma | 1 |
| Myeloma | 1 |
| Aneurysmal bone cyst | 2 |
| Total | 25 |
| Followed | 22 |

**Table 2.** Shoulder Tumor Prostheses (n = 68)

| Metastases from | |
|---|---|
| Breast tumor | 22 |
| Hypernephroma | 12 |
| Thyroid carcinoma | 5 |
| Bronchial carcinoma | 3 |
| Grawitz's tumor | 1 |
| Total | 43 |
| Followed | 36 |

**Table 3.** Shoulder Tumor Prostheses (n = 68)

| Complications | |
|---|---|
| None | 44 |
| Necrotic wound margins | 4 |
| Nerve lesion | 2 |
| Hematoma | 8 |
| Infection | 3 |
| Dislocation | 6 |
| Humeral fracture | 4 |
| Total in 24 patients | 27 |

**Table 4.** Shoulder Tumor Prostheses (n = 58)

| *Subjective result* | |
|---|---|
| Very good | 10 |
| Good | 31 |
| Fair | 13 |
| Poor | 4 |
| *Complaints* | |
| None | 22 |
| Mild | 18 |
| Moderate | 15 |
| Severe | 3 |

**Table 5.** Shoulder Tumor Prostheses (n = 58)

| Postoperative range of motion | Mean | Minimum | Maximum |
|---|---|---|---|
| Elevation | 62.4° | 0° | 160° |
| Abduction | 51.6° | 0° | 125° |
| Internal rotation | 46.4° | 0° | 90° |
| External rotation | 32.6° | 0° | 90° |

giant-cell tumors (8); 1 patient had a spindle-cell sarcoma, and 1 had a myeloma. Our earlier series (collective study) additionally included two cases in which resection was done for an aneurysmal bone cyst - a questionable indication (Table 1).

The majority of metastatic tumors were from breast carcinoma (22), followed by hypernephroma (12), thyroid carcinoma (5), bronchial carcinoma (3), (Fig. 3) and Grawitz's tumor (1). Thirty-six of these patients presented for follow-up (Table 2).

In accordance with the difficulty of the procedure and the patients' initial status, 27 complications arose in 24 patients. The most frequent complication was hematoma (8 cases), followed by dislocation (6), necrotic wound margins (4), humeral fractures (4), and nerve injuries (2). Two patients developed infections (Table 3). The subjective result was good to very good in 41 of 58 patients, fair in 13, and poor in 4. Complaints were absent in 22 patients, minimal in 18, moderate in 15, and severe in 3 (Table 4). Postoperative ranges of motion are shown in Table 5. The mean values

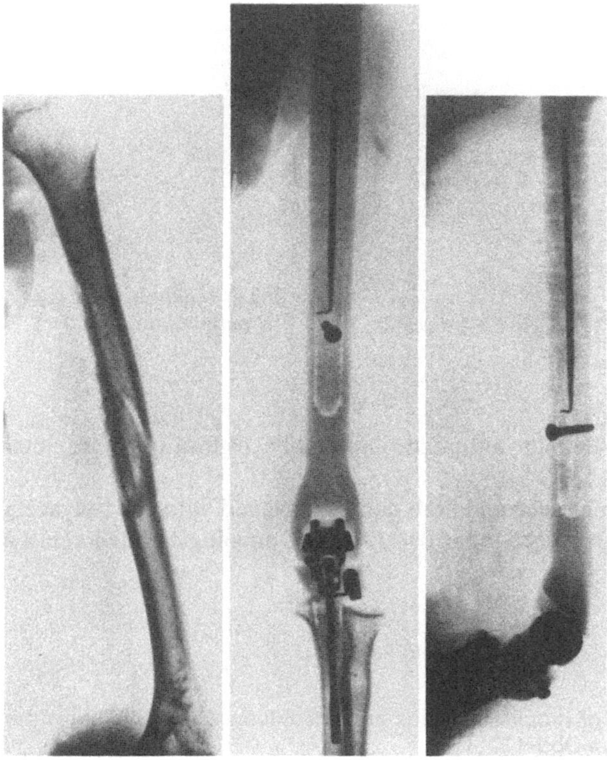

**Fig. 3.** Total humeral replacement for a solitary metastasis from bronchial carcinoma

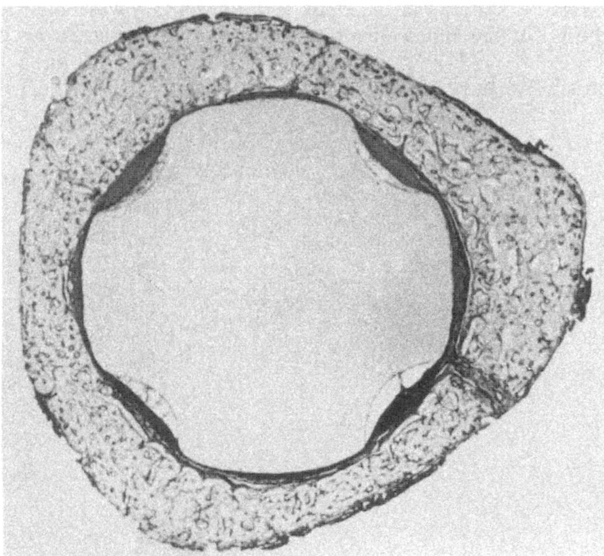

**Fig. 4.** Histologic section at the level of the prosthetic stem 18 months after insertion of a tumor prosthesis

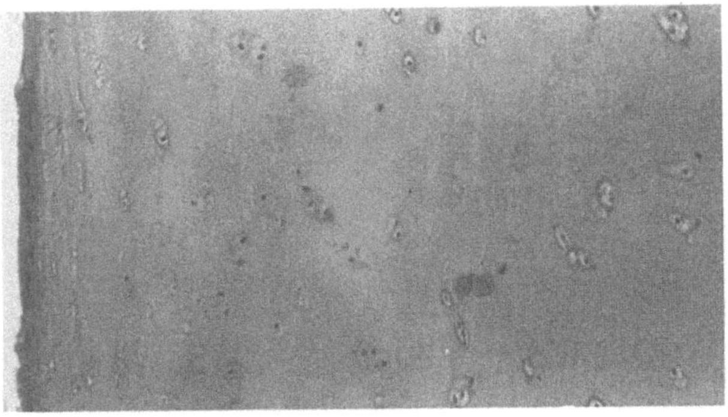

**Fig. 5.** Glenoid cartilage from the same shoulder

showed significant function deficits, although remarkably large values were noted in some individuals.

The results indicate that a serviceable limb can be salvaged with the polyacetal resin tumor prosthesis when it is used in properly selected oncologic patients (Fig. 4, 5).

## References

1. Albee FH (1929) Restoration of shoulder function in cases of loss of head and upper portion of humerus. Surg Gynecol Obstet 32: 1
2. Burri C, Rüter A (1977) Prothesen und Alternativen am Arm. Huber, Bern Stuttgart Wien
3. Burri C, Betzler M (1977) Knochentumoren. Huber, Bern Stuttgart Wien
4. Mathys R (1973) Stand der Verwendung von Kunststoffen für künstliche Gelenke. Aktuel Traumatol 3: 253
5. Salzer M, Knahr K, Locke H, Stärk N, Matejowsky Z, Plenk H jr, Punzei G, Zweymüller K (1979) Bioceramic endoprosthesis for the replacement of the proximal humerus. Arch Orthop Trauma Surg 93: 169
6. Venable CS (1952) Shoulder prosthesis. Am J Surg 83: 271

## Discussion

*Chairman to Sekera:* Problems from traction on the plexus and neurovascular bundle have frequently been reported after the Tikhor-Linberg resection. Has this complaint occurred in any of your patients?

*Sekera:* No.

*Polster:* In very short distal humeral stumps, say 5-7 cm, we have seen cases where the fixation screws broke out of the bone. So we have started reinforcing the fixation with a cemented titanium pin.

*Burri:* A fixation system similar to the fusion pin would probably be best. A cementless implantation is very elegant, but I agree that there is justification for using cement after very long resections.

*Polster:* In our judgment, the subjective assessment of functional results by the patients is of little value, because the patients are faced with a life-threatening situation. Because this procedure salvages the hand, practically all patients will say that they are "satisfied."

*Burri:* I would agree with that statement.

*Polster:* In patients with multifocal metastases and a short life expectancy, we perform a more extensive procedure in order to preserve the function of the hand for that period, although the overall function of the arm is not very satisfactory.

*Knahr:* I would like to ask Dr. Burri how many of his 25 primary tumor resections were "marginal" and how many were "wide." We have been able to achieve wide resections in only a small percentage of our osteosarcoma and chondrosarcoma cases. I also have a question on patient selection: You used prostheses to treat 8 giant-cell tumors and 2 aneurysmal bone cysts. It has been our experience that an equally good result can be obtained by local curettage and bone grafting. As for the total humeral replacement for a metastasis from bronchial carcinoma: Wouldn't this patient have been better off with a composite internal fixation?

*Burri:* That is the treatment we used for that patient, and that certainly could be a matter for discussion.

What we have not observed, unlike yourself, is involvement of the rotator cuff. There were only two cases in which we had to resect the rotator cuff and capsule to obtain adequate surgical margins.

I cannot say much about the results, because we included these 25 patients in the series of 76 cases from 30 centers. Of our own cases, I can tell you that two patients with osteogenic sarcomas have died, and that only one patient with chondrosarcoma has died.

With regard to the aneurysmal bone cysts, these, too, were not our own cases. But as for the giant-cell tumors, I would advise strongly against the local excision of grade II and grade III lesions. Of 537 bone tumors in the German ASIF registry, 37 were classified as semimalignant, and 5 of these patients died within 5 years. Three of them had giant-cell tumors.

*Lettin:* I would like to describe briefly the results of the Royal National Orthopedic Hospital in London, which go back 30 years. The use of prostheses for tumors was introduced by my predecessor, Jackson Burroughs. I personally have not done much work in the area of tumors.

One experience we have had with more than 200 hinged knee prostheses, 17 of which were inserted from 1953 to 1970 and the rest thereafter, is that only 3 have become loose. We have observed that, especially with the titanium prostheses, the intramedullary stems tend to break at the site where the prosthesis seats against the end of the bone. This has been a more frequent complication than loosening of the cement. The cause lies in the better bone quality of the younger tumor patients.

Most of our cases of giant-cell tumors and chondrosarcomas involved the humerus. We always performed the resection just proximal to the deltoid insertion, regardless of X-ray findings, unless it was apparent that the tumor had spread farther distally. Thus, we always sacrificed the rotator cuff and had no problems inserting a prosthesis, although upward subluxation does occur.

*Cofield:* I do not work much with tumors, either, because other colleagues in our group handle that aspect. As much as we like prostheses for these indications, we now do more arthrodeses when the scapula is intact, using massive homologous bone grafts and the ASIF technique of internal fixation. We then place a pedicled fibular graft medially that extends from viable scapula distally to viable humerus. The functional result is that of an arthrodesis, which certainly is not bad in these situations. The cosmetic result is excellent because of the large volume of grafted bone.

Another point should be considered: At our facility (Mayo Clinic) we have hesitated to offer patients chemotherapy, because our results without chemotherapy are almost as good as with it. Moreover, routine chemotherapy would delay healing.

*Sekera:* There is no point to chemotherapy for chondrosarcoma, of course, but it still is appropriate for osteogenic sarcoma. I think that distinction should be made.

When we look at shoulder prostheses that have been in place for 15 years and see that the prosthesis is scarcely distinguishable from bone and that the patients have rotational movement, we become reluctant to sacrifice that function when we do not have to.

In cases where sufficient muscular function can be preserved, we prefer a prosthesis over an arthrodesis. But if the surgery requires sacrifice of the biceps along with the deltoid, we perform an arthrodesis and combine it with a pectoral transfer to the elbow to replace the biceps. This results in reasonably good function of the extremity.

# Stabilization of Shoulders with Bone and Muscle Defects

R. Kölbel

*Suspension* of the hanging and swinging arm during stance and gait and *movement* and *stabilization* of the actively employed arm are essential functions of the shoulder that are disrupted when there is loss of the bony joint members or of the moving and stabilizing muscles about the shoulder.

Below we shall consider these functions, their disturbances, and the effects of those disturbances. Then we shall present clinical examples of techniques that we use to stabilize shoulders with bone and muscle defects.

The structures which stabilize the hanging arm at the shoulder are, in order of importance:

- the muscles
- the capsule and ligaments
- atmospheric pressure (Fig. 1 a).

If the muscular stabilizers are lost (as by paralysis in hemiplegia), a downward subluxation of the humeral head usually develops over a period of about three weeks. This observation shows that when muscular innervation is lost, the joint capsule and ligaments, together with atmospheric pressure, are initially able to maintain glenohumeral reduction against the downward pull of gravity. The capsule is very thin superiorly and posteriorly. It is reinforced in its stabilizing action by the tendons of the supraspinatus and infraspinatus muscles. The anterior part of the capsule is very strong but normally acts only during external rotation and abduction to stabilize the shoulder against displacement anteriorly and to a lesser extent inferiorly.

The superior glenohumeral ligament and coracohumeral ligament are the only parts of the capsule that can prevent downward subluxation of the humerus. They are capable of doing this for only a limited period of time, as the occurrence of subluxation after three weeks demonstrates.

Downward subluxation after fractures of the humeral head also illustrates the importance of the muscular stabilizers, which are lost after trauma due to nociceptive inhibition.

When there is congenital or acquired laxity of the capsule, downward subluxation at the shoulder can be prevented by intact muscular function. Occasionally this leads to static overloading and associated complaints in the muscular stabilizers.

In cases where reduction is not maintained by the joint members, the capsule, or by the joint-spanning muscles, other soft tissues must assume the function of suspending and stabilizing the arm against gravity. These would consist of scars, the neurovascular bundle, and the skin. The results are pain and function impairment involving the neurovascular bundle. Complaints of this type are familiar sequelae to extensive tumor resections about the shoulder which preserve the extremity (Tikhor-Linberg procedure) (Fig. 2 a-d).

Movement of the humerus relative to the scapula follows the principle of the single-arm lever. This presumes that the glenohumeral joint is stabilized and guided by the rotators (Fig. 1 b).

Shoulder Replacement
Eds.: Kölbel/Helbig/Blauth

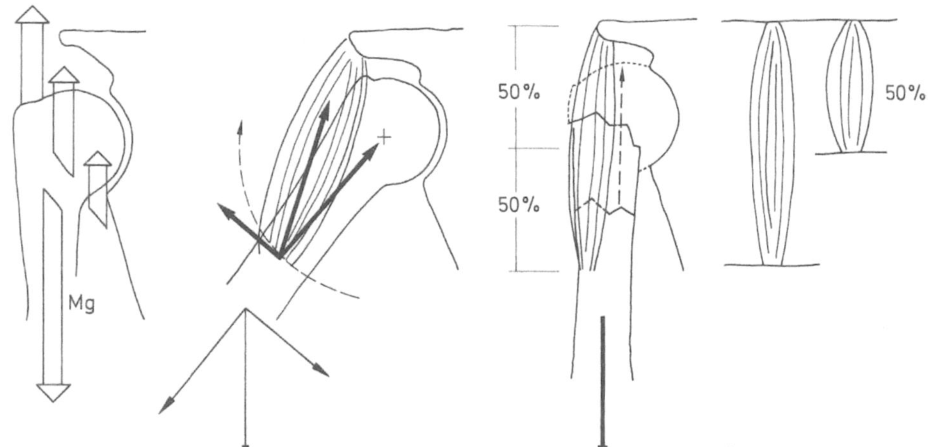


**Fig. 1. a** Suspension of the arm at the shoulder by muscles, capsule, ligaments, and atmospheric pressure. **b** Single-arm lever, components of abducting muscles and segmental weight. **c** When part of the joint is lost (lat. fulcrum) along with part of the suspension, the humerus will tend to displace upward as muscular forces are applied. *Fm* Muscular force; *Mg* weight of segment. **d** The muscle can shorten up to 50% of its length. As the muscle shortens, the force exerted approaches 0%. Loss of bone length = loss of force

This arrangement determines the angular movement of the humerus. The force of the deltoid muscle has one component which acts in the direction necessary for the movement, i.e., perpendicular to the long axis of the humerus and tangential to the arc of motion that is described. This component moves the humerus. The second component must act in the direction of the humerus. (There is no other structure that could transmit the force; only normal forces may be transferred within the joint itself.)

This system works only as long as a functioning joint is present. The moving component can exist only in the presence of a component acting in the longitudinal direction.

When a stable joint is absent, the forces of muscular contraction displace the humerus until the segmental center of gravity is below the point of suspension (Fig. 1 c). When the proximal end of the humerus is lost and the deltoid is intact, the force of the deltoid is greater than the weight of the limb and moves the proximal humerus upward as far as the muscle is able to contract. If the loss of bone length is less than 50% of the muscle length, the proximal end of the humerus is able to engage against the scapula and form a "joint." The residual shortening capacity of the muscle then determines the amount of movement that is possible from that position; i.e., the range of movement and force will be markedly limited (Fig. 1 d). This explains why the active range of motion and force are diminished after a proximal humeral resection or resection arthroplasty, and why a direct relationship exists between loss of bone length and loss of function. In theory, the resection arthroplasty can function only if the deltoid insertion is transposed distally by an amount equal to the length of the proximal bone resection.

There are two reasons, then, for stabilizing a shoulder with bone and muscle defects:

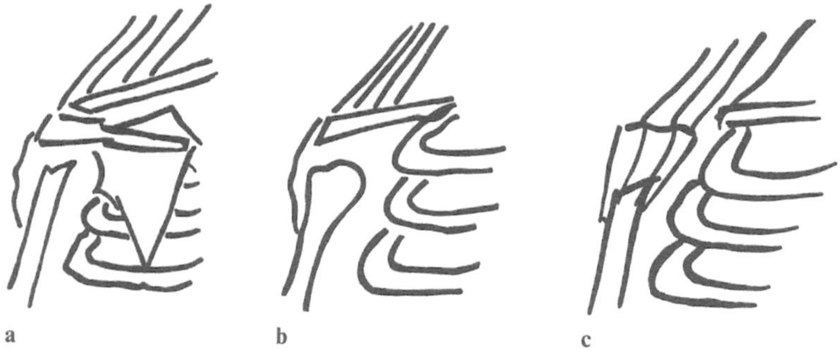

Fig. 2a-c. Shoulder instability after joint resection for various procedures. a Humeral head resection. b Scapulectomy. c Tikhor-Linberg resection

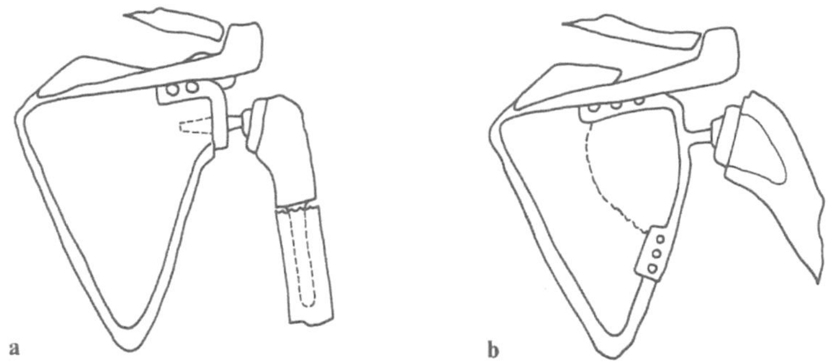

Fig. 3a,b. Constrained implant, modified for use with a humeral defect and for cases requiring scapular reconstruction

1. The suspension of the limb is deficient.
2. The remaining muscles (if present) cannot function without a joint; this applies not just to the deltoid and rotators but also to the thoracohumeral muscles.

Another reason would be cosmesis in cases where stabilization would significantly improve the appearance of the shoulder after an extensive resection of, say, the scapula.

Whether these reasons justify a major operation and, if so, whether one should use a constrained or unconstrained implant will not be considered here. There are several factors that would favor prosthetic surgery, such as immediate stability and shorter postoperative care. With neoplasms, the attempt to salvage the limb must not compromise the objective of adequate tumor control.

I expect that adjuvant chemotherapy will make it possible to attempt limb-salvaging operations with greater frequency, and that implants and anchoring techniques will become better with passage of time.

When faced with a shoulder that has bone and muscle losses but cannot be stabilized with a humeral head prosthesis, I use a stable, constrained prosthesis whose mode of attachment to cortical structures of the scapula has proven very successful clinically. In almost all cases, the device had to be individually modified (Fig. 3a,b).

My experience with six patients is outlined below:

*Case 1*

The implant was first used in a 74-year-old woman with painful instability after resection of the humeral head. Only the spinal part and some of the acromial part of the deltoid were preserved. The patient was satisfied with the functional result for five years. In the sixth year the joint, which she used as an arthrodesis to rotate the shoulder into abduction, dislocated upon lifting a heavy load. At reoperation, the scapular component was found to be solidly attached (Fig. 4 a-d).

*Case 2*

A similar situation existed in a 76-year-old woman after humeral head resection for a nonunion, attempted prosthetic replacement, and a failed Putti-Platt procedure to stabilize for subluxation. Pain was the major reason for stabilizing this patient with a modified implant.

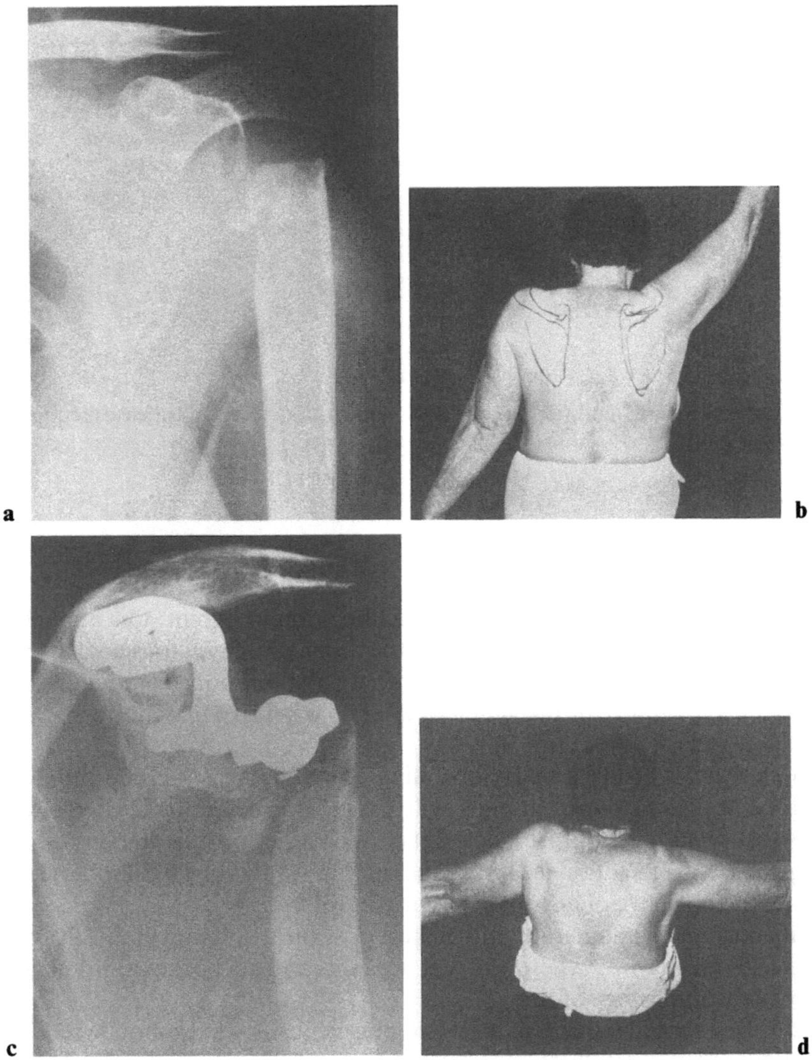


**Fig. 4 a-d.** Shoulder with bone and muscle defects after humeral head resection in a 74-year-old woman. Radiographic appearance and function in 5th postoperative year, about 1 year prior to dislocation of the joint. A fragment of the metal retaining ring is visible. (Left side operated)

Fracture of the osteoporotic humerus was predictable, and so we prepared a humeral component with an elongated metal stem. At five years postoperatively the patient is satisfied with the result. She has some discomfort in the area of the trapezius insertion when a heavy coat is worn (Fig. 5 a,b).

*Case 3*

In a 64-year-old woman with a very painful metastasis from a medullary carcinoma, we elected to replace the upper third of the humerus with a modified implant. The patient was free of pain and survived for six months. In this case the axillary nerve had been sacrificed at tumor resection.

*Case 4*

Resection of the upper half of the humerus was indicated in a man about 40 years of age with a malignant fibrous histiocytoma. The humeral component of the constrained implant was modified by utilizing a ceramic stem. The operation was performed at Ehime University by Prof. Shibata. The result according to the latest report at 7 months postoperatively was excellent according to Enneking's criteria.

In the cases described above, it was necessary to bridge an osseous defect of the humerus. In the cases that follow, the scapula was damaged by the tumor, and it was necessary to bridge the scapular defect or to stabilize the residual scapula. In both cases it was found that the remaining portion of the scapula was very unstable after the partial scapulectomy. The scapula is a framelike structure that receives and transmits muscular forces. If the frame becomes disrupted at any point, the system loses rigidity. Thus, in arthroplasty one is concerned not just with achieving fixation of the joint implant but also with restoring scapular stability.

*Case 5*

A 56-year-old woman had an osteolytic lesion of the scapular neck and glenoid that was metastatic to thyroid carcinoma. This was the only metastasis known to be present. Radiotherapeutic options were exhausted, and further radiotherapy was rejected by the radiotherapist, who suggested surgical resection.

The base of the scapular spine was still intact. The implant was supplemented with an out-

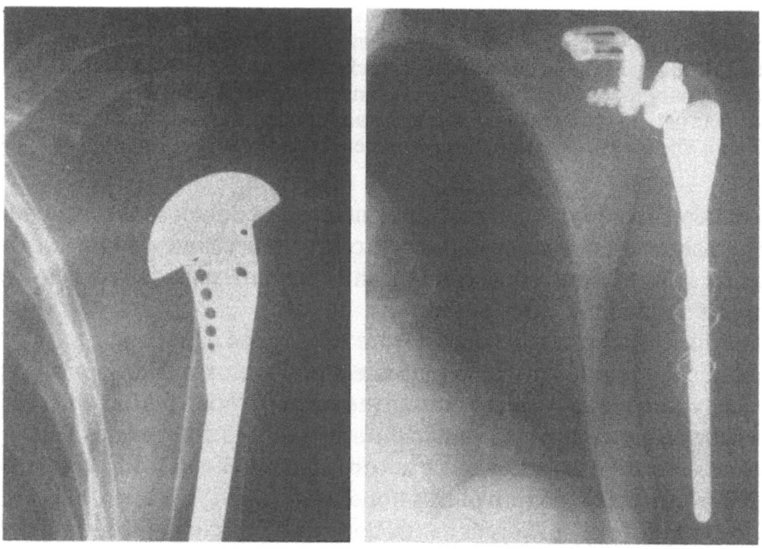

a b

**Fig. 5 a,b.** Woman 76 years of age with osseous defect of proximal humerus and shortening after reoperation (Putti-Platt), before and after stabilization

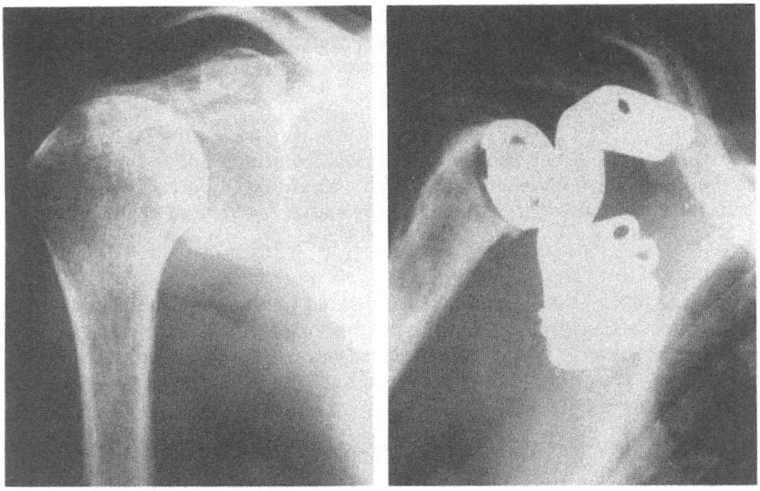
a b

**Fig. 6a,b.** Woman 56 years of age with solitary metastasis from thyroid carcinoma. Radiographs before and after resection and stabilization with a constrained implant that reconstructs the scapula

rigger for fixation to the lateral margin. The tumor resection required sacrifice of the nerve branch to the infraspinatus, which was involved by tumor. The scapular component was attached to the cortical structures with screws. The patient was free of pain and satisfied with her function until 2 years and 6 months later, when a scapulectomy had to be performed because of a local recurrence. The scapular component of the implant was still solidly attached to the bone on the surgical specimen (Fig. 6 a,b).

*Case 6*
A 54-year-old man had a long-standing chondrosarcoma of the left scapula involving the glenoid, scapular neck, coracoid process, and body of the scapula. The tumor was resected with a soft tissue margin of about 2 cm, requiring sacrifice of adjacent muscles and the suprascapular nerve. Again, a modified scapular component was used. The remaining base of the spine was just wide enough to accommodate three screws. The remainder of the scapula was very unstable, and the body of the scapula became cracked. Attachment of the scapular component to the lateral margin and base of the spine reconstructed the frame of the scapula and restored stability. The patient was free of complaints, and function was satisfactory, as we had expected (Fig. 7 a-e). The patient died with extensive metastasis 1 year and 6 months postoperatively.

Both of these patients required muscle advancements to maintain serviceable muscle lengths. The patients did not develop infections or other complications. However, the outcomes demonstrate that caution and restraint are advised when attempting to restore function in cases of this type.

The following conclusions may be drawn from our limited experience:

1. Besides stabilizing the shoulder with replacement of the proximal humerus, it appears technically feasible also to reconstitute the scapula with a partial prosthesis.
2. Experience with fixation of this implant to the scapula in 18 other cases over a period of 10 years indicates that attachment to cortical parts of the scapula is particularly useful for the reconstruction of this bone.
3. Functional expectations in a shoulder with bone and muscle defects should remain realistic, even when a constrained prosthesis is used.
4. Improvements in operating technique appear possible.

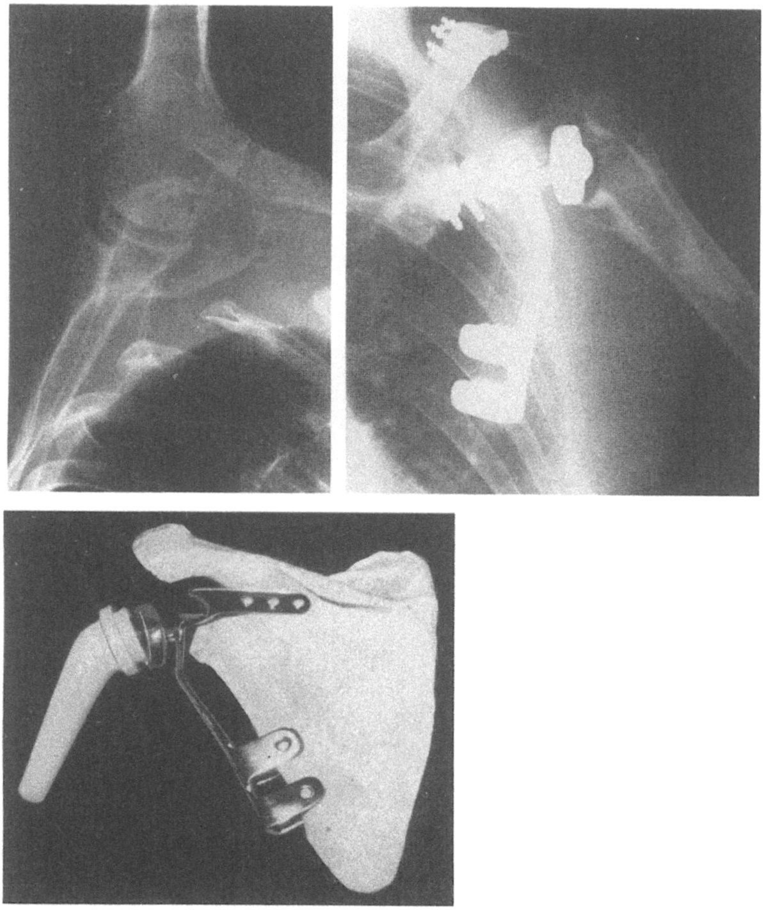

a c b

**Fig. 7 a-c.** Man 54 years of age with chondrosarcoma of the coracoid process involving the neck and body of the scapula. Preoperative radiograph, implant to stabilize the shoulder and reconstruct the scapula, postoperative radiograph

5. Tumor resection takes precedence over reconstruction.
6. If this rule is respected, there appear to be few objections to using implants in similar cases. A stable shoulder with limited function and all the other limitations of prosthetic replacement is a reasonable alternative to a painful, unstable joint.

Time will tell whether a more ambitious replacement, such as replacement of the entire scapula (Eckardt et al. 1985), is feasible. It is certain that further attempts will be made in that direction.

## References

Eckardt J, Eilber F, Jinnah R (1985) Endoprosthetic replacement of the scapula and shoulder joint for malignant tumors of the scapula. A preliminary report. American Shoulder and Elbow Surgeons, Annual Meeting 1985

# Recent Developments in Shoulder Replacement and Early Results

# Radiographic and Clinical Assessment of the Macnab-English Porous-Coated Total Shoulder Replacement

J. P. McElwain and E. English

## Introduction

The short-term complications associated with prosthetic replacement of the diseased shoulder joint have been documented by a number of investigators including Amstutz, Kessel, Neer, and Post [1, 4-8, 10].

Despite the many types of prosthesis that have been developed, loosening and breakage of the material continue to be major complications. Inadequate periarticular musculature, predominantly in the rotator cuff, has necessitated the use of more constrained prostheses that have a certain amount of intrinsic stability. Constrained prostheses are more susceptible to loosening because of the magnitude of the forces across the glenohumeral anchorage. Incidences of loosening as high as 25% have been reported for the cemented, constrained types like the Stanmore prosthesis [7, 10]. Given this unacceptably high loosening rate, alternative sources of fixation must be sought.

Over the last decade, attention has been given to biologic fixation by bone and fibrous tissue ingrowth into porous-coated implants made of different types of material. It has been shown experimentally by Cameron and Pilliar [2, 3, 9] that biologic fixation does occur with successful implantation, depending on the presence of minimal tissue-implant movement, a press-fit of the implant to healthy cancellous bone, and suitable pore size, presently considered to be in the range of 50 to 400 um.

Radiographic findings in experimental animals include bone resorption due to stress protection, and radiolucent lines in close proximity to the implants, which are thought to be due to micromotion. It is recognized that differentiation between fibrous and bony ingrowth is difficult in the absence of histologic specimens.

The main purpose of this evaluation is to review the earliest cases of the English-Macnab porous-coated total shoulder replacement, with special emphasis placed on radiographic features.

The prosthesis was introduced for a limited clinical trial in 1976. It is essentially an unconstrained prosthesis in which stability is enhanced by a superior hood or ledge that projects over the top of a small portion of the humeral head. This ledge provides additional stability in the event the rotator cuff is diseased or nonfunctional.

A glenoid component is available that is metal-backed and has a porous coating. The idea of this design is to allow tissue ingrowth into the metal-backed base. The glenoid component can be fitted with an optional acromial arm that extends up to the acromion for added stability. This is used only if the rotator cuff is absent. Medium and long acromial pins are present to counteract rotation and improve stability. Orthochrome screws are used to anchor the glenoid to the bone for short-term stability while tissue ingrowth occurs. An ultrahigh-molecular-weight polyethylene insert snaps into the glenoid component to provide low-friction articulation for the humeral head (Fig. 1).

Shoulder Replacement
Eds.: Kölbel/Helbig/Blauth

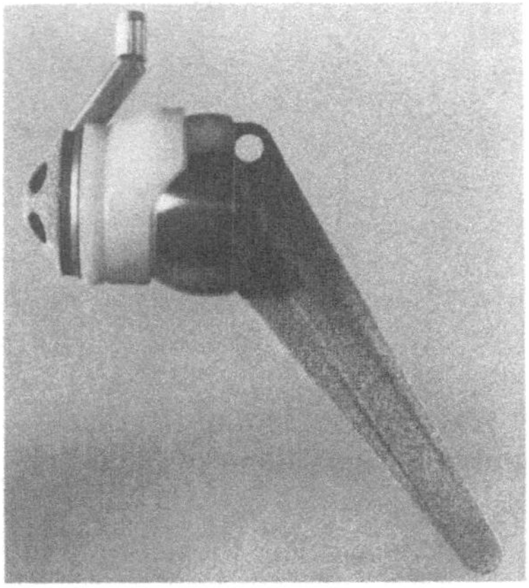

**Fig. 1.** Porous-coated shoulder prosthesis with acromial arm

At present two sizes of humeral stems are available, the narrower stem being reserved for patients with narrow medullary cavities. The stems are porous-coated over their entire length. The pore sizes for both components range from 150 to 400 μm.

Each prosthesis is designed to allow 110° of glenohumeral motion on both the sagittal and coronal planes. The head size with its corresponding glenoid component has been designed to reestablish the normal shoulder position and movement.

## Materials

Twenty-one porous-coated total shoulder arthroplasties have been performed since the start of the clinical trial. Analysis of the clinical results and radiographic findings is presented here for 13 of the patients. Five of the 21 patients died, and 3 were lost to follow-up. The small number of patients in this series demonstrates the high selectivity of the patients for the operation. The authors felt that this type of arthroplasty should not be done on a regular basis until long-term follow-ups are able to demonstrate the reliability of porous coating. The average age of the patients was 62 years (46-81 years). The average follow-up was 37 months. The preoperative diagnosis was osteoarthritis secondary to trauma or primary osteoarthritis in six patients, rheumatoid arthritis in five patients, villonodular synovitis in one patients, and psoriatic arthritis in one patient.

Only patients with severe arthropathy were considered candidates for total shoulder replacement. Surgery was considered only after all forms of conservative management had failed. The main indication for surgery was intractable pain due to incongruity of the glenoid and humeral head. In recommending surgery, we advised all patients about the unpredictable improvement in range of motion and function. The primary objective was to eliminate pain. Motion was a secondary concern. All patients had significantly weakened function because of joint incongruity and rotator cuff involvement. All patients with rheumatoid arthritis had a significantly decreased functional capacity of the rotator cuff muscles.

Serial AP, lateral, and transaxillary radiographs were studied for changes in the humerus and glenoid. Standard radiographic views were difficult to reproduce following shoulder arthroplasty, but it was possible in nearly all cases to make direct comparisons. The interfaces between the implant and bone were evaluated for loosening, remodeling, resorption, cancellous new bone formation, humeral prosthetic subsidence, prosthetic shifting, and radiopaque zones surrounding the prosthesis. The relationship of the humeral head to the glenoid was also assessed.

## Radiographic Findings

On the humeral side, most of the changes occurred proximally. The features recognized were, in order of frequency, resorption of the proximal medial cortex (9 patients), prosthetic subsidence (7 patients), cancellous new bone formation (7 patients), proximal humeral remodeling (5 patients), and prosthetic shifting (1 patient) (Figs. 2 and 3).

Resorption of the proximal cortex was commonly seen between three and six months, appearing as early as two months in one case. The amount of resorption never exceeded 6 mm and seemed to relate to the activity of the patient. It was usually seen in cases where there was not sufficient contact between the prosthesis and proximal humerus, implying little if any stress transfer in that area.

Proximal humeral remodeling was noted most often when there was less than adequate contact between the prosthesis and the medial side of the humerus. Shifting of the prosthetic stem within the medullary cavity occurred in one patient; we now consider this to be an indication of loosening. A change in the position of the humeral stem is difficult to document, since it depends on such variables as humeral rotation and image magnification. It is possible that shifting occurred in two other patients, as evidenced by the presence of radiolucent lines.

In one patient we saw a radiopaque line located a constant distance from the humeral implant and extending the whole length of the prosthesis. In a second patient we saw a similar line around only the lower third and tip of the prosthesis. In one case these lines were visible at 12 months in a patient who had received a smaller implant. It was initially seen on the sagittal plane and may relate to movement of the prosthesis within the medullary cavity during forward flexion due to malalignment of the prosthesis and an improper press-fit between the prosthesis and bone. Both patients with radiopaque lines are asymptomatic at one year and three years, respectively. The lines are similar in appearance to those described experimentally by Pilliar [9]. He considers these lines to represent hypertrophic cancellous bone separated from the implant by a thin layer of fibrous tissue whose fibers are arranged obliquely. In humans, the exact significance of these radiopaque lines in unclear. The difference between the radiopaque lines seen around porous-coated implants and nonporous-coated implants is illustrated in our experience with the nonporous-coated prosthesis. There is a wider interval of lucency, and the radiopaque line, though not well defined, occurs at a more constant distance from the surface of the nonporous-coated implant.

Cancellous new bone formation is difficult to quantify, because even slight changes in radiographic density and position will alter the X-ray appearance. We were able to identify new cancellous bone on the medial aspect and to a lesser extent the lateral aspect of the proximal humerus in seven of our patients. This implies that compressive forces are being transferred to the bone in this area.

Remodeling around the glenoid, predominantly on the superior and inferior sur-

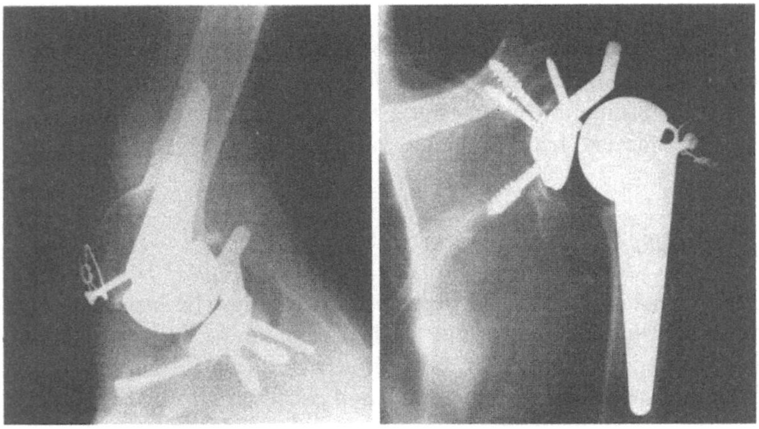

**Fig. 2.** Shoulder prosthesis with nonpainful glenoid lucencies

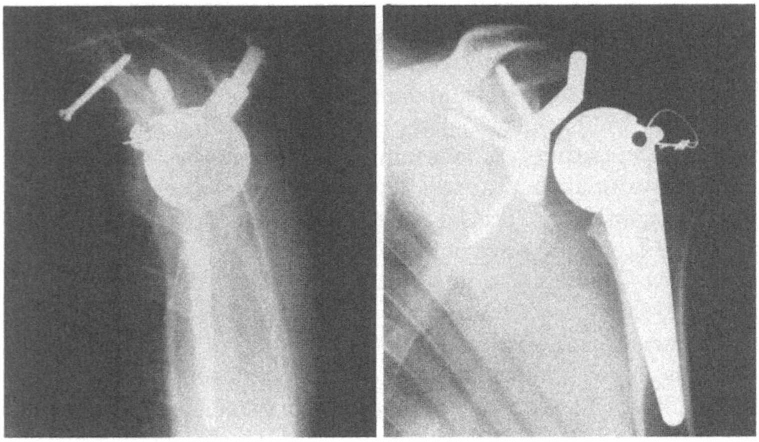

**Fig. 3.** Shoulder prosthesis with adaptive changes in the humerus: cancellous new bone formation on the shaft and neck

faces, was evident in five patients. There was considerable lucency surrounding one glenoid component. This component was considered to be loose. Close inspection of the remaining seven showed good fixation without obvious adaptive changes. Radiopaque lines like those seen in the humeral diaphysis were not visible in the glenoid. There was no evidence of implant shifting. Areas of lucency surrounding the anchoring screws were noted in a number of cases. Migration of the glenoid component was documented in these cases, but all the patients were clinically asymptomatic.

The relationship of the head to the glenoid was studied to evaluate the amount of proximal migration. Because of the variation in positions on serial radiographs, only films that showed obvious migration were considered. Aside from one patient with persistent anterior subluxation, only three patients had significant humeral migration, and all three had totally deficient rotator cuffs.

## Clinical Results

The clinical results were evaluated using a modification of the University of California at Los Angeles shoulder rating system reported by Amstutz in 1981 [1]. Activities of daily living, with particular reference to personal care, were also recorded.

Overall improvement in pain relief was satisfactory in 11 of 13 patients. At follow-up seven had no pain, four had slight pain not requiring analgesia, and two had moderate to severe pain, one due to glenoid loosening and the other to persitent anterior subluxation.

Improvement in function was confirmed in all but two patients and was best in individuals with good musculature. Overall functional improvement in patients with rheumatoid arthritis was compromised by the absence of the rotator cuff and by the progression of disease in other joints of the upper limbs. Perineal hygiene was improved in 11 of 13 patients, and 8 patients could comb their hair. Range of motion was improved in seven, unchanged in two, and decreased in four.

Forward flexion averaged 57° preoperatively and 84° postoperatively. Only two patients had forward flexion greater than 100°. The average range of postoperative abduction was 56°. The main component was scapulothoracic movement with minimal glenohumeral abduction and forward flexion, but with reasonably good rotation at the glenohumeral joint. Marginal improvement in rotation without pain was very satisfying to most patients.

## Complications

Radiographic evidence of humeral component loosening was noted in one patient at two years postoperatively, despite a relative absence of symptoms. This patient has a good functional result, has no loss of bone stock, and revision is not contemplated at this time. One dislocation occurred at seven months, and this patient went on to develop a loose glenoid. It is possible that the glenoid was loose from the outset. Revision was considered unwise.

A segmental fracture of the humeral shaft surrounding the prosthesis resulted from a fall in one patient 3 1/2 years following replacement. Fixation of the fracture was effected with Partridge plates and bands. These resulted in excessive bone resorption due to stress shielding. The radiographic features now suggest loosening, which was not present prior to the fracture. Loosening of the glenoid plastic insert occurred in one patient. This patient now has a persistent anterior subluxation following revision of the plastic insert. Fatigue fracture of the orthochrome screws occurred twice but did not compromise the glenoid fixation. Most of these complications, which are due to technical imperfections, occurred during the early stage of the clinical trial and have not been experienced since that time.

## Discussion

Successful documentation of these subtle X-ray changes requires an accurate radiographic technique. It entails proper patient positioning with correct rotational positioning of the humerus for each successive evaluation. The tube, shoulder, and cassette distance must be kept constant to prevent undesired image magnification.

Similar exposures must be used for all examinations, and the intervals between examinations should be constant.

In this series we are able to comment only on the presence or progression of adaptive changes seen on standard, comparable radiographic views. Obtaining standard views of the humerus with exact rotation depends initially on the stage of rehabilitation of the patient and later on the residual mobility of the shoulder. It is extremely difficult to obtain a true radiograph of the glenoid component in a patient with poor shoulder function.

Adaptive changes were observed more frequently in patients with improved shoulder function. It is possible that relative inactivity due to muscular weakness accounted for the relative lack of adaptive changes seen in patients with rheumatoid arthritis. Sufficient fixation of the implant by bone or fibrous tissue ingrowth was obtained in 12 humeri and 12 glenoids with an average follow-up of 3 years. Although one humeral component is radiographically loose, it is not causing pain. The patient with the loose glenoid has pain requiring analgesic medication. Two patients with radiopaque lines around the humeral component are pain-free, indicating that sufficient fixation has taken place. Overall function improved in all patients but two. Range-of-motion improvement was variable and seemed to relate to the condition of the surrounding soft tissues (especially the rotator cuff muscles), the patient's general condition relative to the underlying disease process, and the chronicity of the preoperative disease.

In all cases it was not possible to differentiate between fibrous and bony ingrowth, but the clinical results and observations suggest that the prostheses were not loose, and that there was no radiographic or clinical deterioration over time. Postmortem retrieval of these prostheses has not been possible in the five patients who died.

An average follow-up of three years is not sufficient to assess the durability of this system. But given the degree of fixation and the level of clinical improvement, we feel confident that further clinical use of this prosthesis is justified for selected patients with arthritis of the shoulder. The procedure is difficult, and attention to technical details is important if mechanical complications are to be avoided.

## Summary

A clinical trial of total shoulder replacement with porous-coated implants has been undertaken over the last six years. A limited number of patients have been followed and reviewed for at least three years after their primary surgery. It is difficult to determine whether stability was obtained by fibrous or bony tissue ingrowth into the prosthesis, or by a combination of both. With the exception of two patients (one glenoid and one humeral component), there was no obvious radiographic evidence of loosening. The clinical results were variable. Long-term evaluation is necessary, but the early follow-up is encouraging.

## References


1. Amstutz AC, Sew Hoy AL, Clark RC (1981) UCLA anatomic total shoulder arthroplasty. Clin Orthop 155: 7-20
2. Bobyn JD, Cameron HU, Abdulla D, Pilliar RM, Weatherby GC (1982) Biologic fixation and bone remodelling with an unconstrained canine total knee prosthesis. Clin Orthop 166: 301-311
3. Cameron HU, Pilliar RM, MacNab I (1973) The effects of movement on the bonding of porous metal to bone. J Biomed Matter Res 7: 301
4. Clayton ML, Ferlie DC, Jeffers PD (1982) Prosthetic arthroplasties of the shoulder. Clin Orthop 164: 184-191
5. Coughlin MJ, Morris JM, West WF (1979) The semi-constrained total shoulder arthroplasty. J Bone Joint Surg [Am] 61: 574-581
6. Kessel L, Bayley I (1979) Prosthetic replacement of the shoulder joint. Preliminary communication. J R Soc Med 72: 748-752
7. Lettin AWF, Copeland SA, Scales JT (1982) The Stanmore total shoulder replacement. J Bone Joint Surg [Br] 64: 47-51
8. Neer CS, Watson KC, Stanton FJ (1982) Recent experience in total shoulder replacement. J Bone Joint Surg [Am] 64: 319-337
9. Pilliar RM, Cameron HU, Welsh RP, Binnington AG (1981) Radiographic and morphological studies of load bearing porous surfaced structured implants. Clin Orthop 56: 249-257
10. Post M, Haskell SS, Jablon F (1980) Total shoulder replacement with a constrained prosthesis. J Bone Joint Surg [Am] 62: 327-335

# Discussion

*Chairman:* It is my impression that the humeral components became well incorporated. But this is more difficult to assess in the glenoid components. It is reasonable to assume that fixation with screws is effective and necessary if we assume that no bony contact is established with the rough surface coating. I would hope that it will be possible one day to examine an actual specimen so that the amount of bone ingrowth into surface irregularities can be assessed directly.

*N. N.:* What technique do you use to insert the humeral component?

*English:* We use a rasp that is slightly undersized relative to the humeral component. This instrument comes in two sizes at the present time.

*Polster:* The lucent margins that were observed raise the question of migration. Did the glenoid or humeral component become loose? Did you observe migration in specific directions, such as upward or posteriorly?

*English:* If you saw a change in the orientation of the implant on any of the films that were shown, we believe that that indeed was due to migration. But we saw significant shifting in only one glenoid component, and true loosening in only one humeral component. I do not believe that the lucent lines were visible beforehand. There is no relationship between lucent lines and complaints, so I do not believe that this finding necessarily signifies interfacial motion. It more likely represents a compaction of the cancellous bone around the prosthesis, and that is an adaptive change due to remodeling.

*Chairman:* Do you place minimum requirements on the scapula to which the glenoid component is attached?

*English:* I do not believe that a minimum exists. I had two patients with dysplasia, and we used custom-fabricated implants in both cases. The glenoid component is not always fitted completely into the glenoid fossa. I have found that the anterior rim of the glenoid is often heavily eroded, especially in rheumatoid patients, and that the posterior rim is usually intact. I believe that a good press-fit into the reamed cavity with full peripheral contact would be ideal. I have had one case where the anterior rim fractured at operation; I simply left it in alone, and the fracture healed.

*Chairman:* I had thought that the glenoid unit must be supported by at least 3/4 of its circumference in order to get a reliable fixation with screws. Is that true?

*English:* Yes, I believe that the anchorage is stable when at least 3/4 of the glenoid is preserved; it is not always 100%, but it is certainly very stable. At the end of the procedure you can lift the patient from the table by the two Vitallium screws.

*N. N.:* What criteria did you use in determining the placement of the screws?

*English:* We chose this particular screw placement because there is very little bone behind the glenoid fossa. The bone is somewhat thicker below the coracoid, and then there is the lateral margin of the scapula. So we prefer to drive screws into the base of the coracoid process and down into the lateral scapular margin. The baseplate of the glenoid component has four holes that allow correct placement of the screws.

I would like to add that this prosthesis has a ledge at the upper rim of the polyethylene articular surface, which is designed to prevent superior migration of the prosthesis. Except for the one case that I showed you, this kind of migration did not occur.

*Chairman:* How many of your patients had rotator cuff defects, and how many prostheses did you have to stabilize with an acromial arm?

*English:* My original intent was to use the acromial arm in all cases, because I found it necessary to stabilize the shoulder as well as possible for bone ingrowth into the porous surfaces. It has turned out that increasing numbers of our patients have intact rotator cuffs. That was left out in the previous discussion. So we are not talking about cuff-tear arthropathies, which were mentioned this morning, but about osteoarthritis and rheumatoid arthritis. The quality of the rotator cuff is definitely adequate in at least 50% of patients and probably adequate in another 20%. It is totally inadequate in only about 30%.

I initially used abduction pillows and splints for postoperative care. To date I have inserted over 100 prostheses, but here I am reporting only on a relatively small group of cases that have been followed. After I found that bandages and splints prolonged rehabilitation, I followed the example of McNab and used only a sling for the first 2-3 weeks to reduce gravity forces on the shoulder and to alleviate pain. Afterward the arm is not immobilized further. The patient performs active assisted exercises or in some cases passive exercises, depending on his cooperation. We first exercise with gravity suspension and build from there. We use passive exercises as necessary to preserve the passive range of motion; this is especially important in rheumatoids, who usually do not have enough muscular strength to move the shoulder. We maintain passive motion until the muscles are strong enough that the patient can utilize the range of motion that has been achieved.

I should add that I have not mobilized any patients under anesthesia.

*Welsh:* I am very interested in this project, because it is perhaps the first clinical application of a technique that I started in 1969 with a metallurgist, Dr. Pilliar. Dr. English and Dr. Cameron have taken the project a step farther, and Dr. English finally applied it to the shoulder.

In my opinion there is no better fixation of the glenoid component that mechanical fixation with screws. Also, I doubt that the truncated conical shape of the base of the glenoid component provides sufficient bony contact for ingrowth to occur. You may have had few loosenings, but I do not believe that the glenoid is solidly seated.

As for the humeral component, the porous surface may well be receptive to bony ingrowth. If I were to redesign it, I would make stems of varying thicknesses to get a better distal seating; only the proximal part of the stem would need to have a porous coating for bonding with the bone.

Regarding the function of a shoulder with this prosthesis, I am bothered, like many others, by total shoulder implants that do not approximate the range of motion - in flexion - that is possible with plain scapulothoracic movement. I believe that glenohumeral motion is minimal in a number of our prostheses, even the Neer device. What kind of rotation do you obtain with these prostheses? As far as I am concerned, that is really the only functional goal with a total shoulder prosthesis of this type.

*English:* I agree that rotation is the best of the functions that is achieved. That is why I consider total arthroplasty better than an arthrodesis. It enables the patient to reach the hair and also the perineum, which is very difficult with an arthrodesis. I also agree that fixation of the glenoid component is probably a screw fixation, comparable to the acetabular fixation in uncemented hips. I believe that contraction of the shoulder muscles keeps the prosthesis in place where it was inserted.

I would agree with you that shoulder motion is very limited in flexion and abduction. Initially I resected the acromioclavicular joints in all patients in order to improve the range of motion, but this did not succeed. I could achieve no more scapulothoracic movement than nature provided for.

The humeral component is being redesigned at the present time.

*Lettin:* As far as range of motion is concerned, I have no doubt that you can improve glenohumeral flexion and also abduction to some extent. Most of the rheumatoids that I have treated had no preoperative movement in the glenohumeral joint and had flexion of just less than 45° to not quite 60°, but all of them had scapulothoracic motion. The improvement to 90° after surgery shows that the range of motion is doubled by the reestablishment of glenohumeral movement.

Concerning ingrowth, I agree that it is obtainable experimentally - if we extrapolate the primary bone healing seen with stable fixation - but I doubt that it can occur without absolute mechanical rest. This would probably make it very difficult to achieve in the hip and knee. We do not want to subject our patients to 8-12 weeks of non-weight bearing if we can avoid it.

# Total Shoulder Arthroplasty with Bone Ingrowth Fixation

R. H. Cofield

The initial belief that the small amount of bone available in the glenoid for fixation of a prosthetic component would be the limiting factor in total shoulder replacement is probably true. Although failure of total shoulder arthroplasty using the unconstrained devices is infrequent, we anticipate with extension of our current statistics that at least 10% of total shoulder replacements will require reoperation within 5 years after surgery.

There are a number of extrapolations from total joint replacement in the hip and knee that can be applied to the shoulder. Some of these involve prosthetic design and method of use, and others apply to operative technique. Concerning operative technique, it is well recognized that various means can be used to improve the results of cement fixation. The components must be correctly aligned, subchondral bone support should be preserved, and it is desirable to gain cortical support whenever possible. As for the component, prosthetic material selection is an important consideration here as elsewhere. Thin, high-density polyethylene components should be avoided, and metal backing should be used when possible. Many of these concepts developed in other areas have been applied to the shoulder, as illustrated by the new Neer type of glenoid component, which incorporates a metal backing.

One potentially important area of development in the hip and knee that can be applied to the shoulder is the use of materials that are receptive to bone ingrowth. The manufacture of ingrowth materials has become practical from a technical standpoint, and more information is becoming available on optimum pore sizes, the percentage of porosity on the surface, necessary pore depths, and the positioning of the porous surface of the implant.

When designing a porous ingrowth component, we felt very strongly that it should be of the unconstrained type. It should offer the option of use either as a proximal humeral replacement alone or in conjunction with a glenoid component for total shoulder arthroplasty. Also, we felt it highly desirable to design the surface curvature so that it would be compatible with other commonly used unconstrained implants. This would allow some system interchangeability, which is useful during initial surgery and can be especially valuable in revision work. Design features must include adequate primary fixation to permit early postoperative motion at the shoulder, and this would require a tight interference fit that might perhaps be supplemented by anchoring screws. There should also be a reasonable potential for ingrowth when the porous surface is placed in apposition to cancellous or corticocancellous bone.

Figure 1 shows the glenoid component disassembled. The metal tray has porous ingrowth material on its back surface and can accommodate two screws. The high-density polyethylene insert is also shown. Figure 2 shows the polyethylene component positioned in the metal tray. Instrumentation is relatively simple and includes a facing reamer, two templates to allow positioning of the drill holes for the columns, and three drills with different depth markings.

Shoulder Replacement
Eds.: Kölbel/Helbig/Blauth

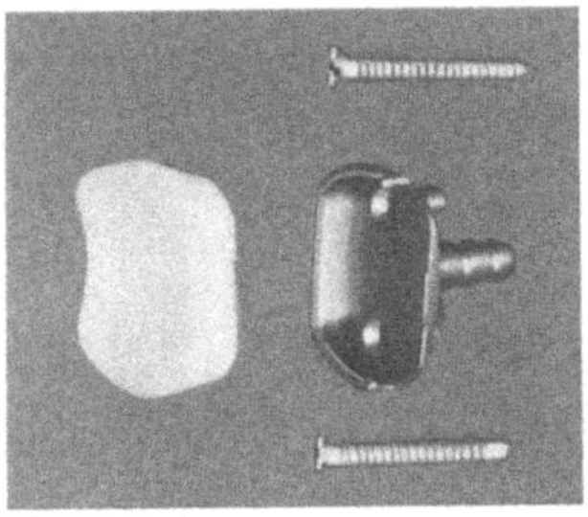

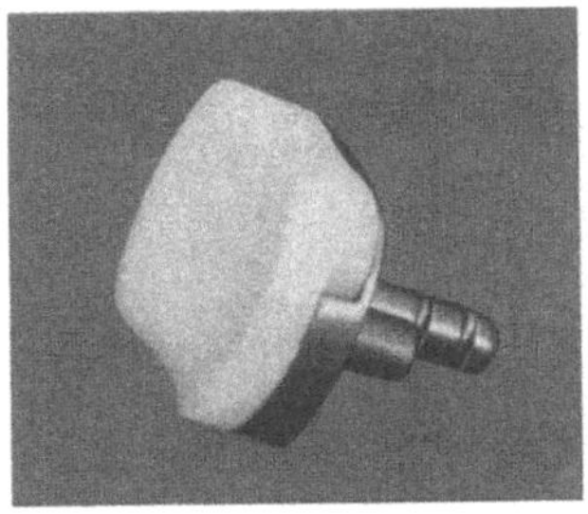

**Fig. 1** **Fig. 2**

**Fig. 1.** A disassembled porous-ingrowth glenoid component. The porous surface is on the back of the metal tray

**Fig. 2.** Polyethylene component positioned in the metal tray

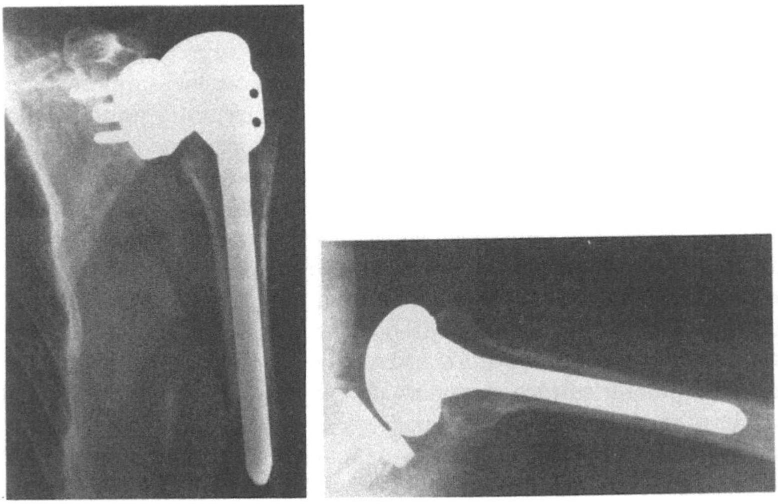

a b

**Fig. 3a,b.** Man 32 years of age with rheumatoid arthritis. The porous-ingrowth components are in place. **a** AP view. **b** Axillary view

Figure 3 shows the postoperative film of a young rheumatoid patient in whom this type of glenoid component was combined with a proximal humeral component with porous ingrowth material on the posterior surface of the head.

Patient selection involves multiple considerations. At present the porous ingrowth implants would seem most appropriate for active individuals, regardless of age. Adequate bone support must be present in terms of volume as well as density, and the patient must understand and accept the potential benefits and somewhat ill-defined risks of this procedure. Our patients who were treated with this prosthesis fell into two groups: those who had cement fixation of the implant to assess the usefulness of the implant per se, and those who had interference and screw fixation to assess 1) the adequacy of the primary fixation and 2) the frequency of ingrowth bonding of the components.

Between March, 1983, and May, 1985, the glenoid component was cemented in 17 shoulders and placed without cement in 21 shoulders so that bone ingrowth could occur. The average age at operation was 66 years in patients with cemented implants and 60 years in patients with uncemented implants. Males predominated in both groups, because only one size of glenoid component was available, and it was medium to medium-large in size. The diagnoses in these patients reflect the diagnostic distribution of our patients in general, and the adjunctive surgical procedures are similar to those used in our more general patient group that has received total shoulder implants.

Follow-up evaluations are, of course, still incomplete at this time. The cemented group was evaluated first, and follow-up is generally in the one- to two-year range. Surgery was more recent in the uncemented group, and so their follow-up is from six months to one year.

Analysis of pain has been quite easy. All patients had moderate or severe pain preoperatively, and postoperative pain relief has been satisfactory in all cases.

Motion is difficult to analyze at this point, since rehabilitation is incomplete. As expected, the gains in rotation have come early in the postoperative period, while gains in upward movement with return of strength occur at a slower pace.

Two patients had rotator cuff retearing in the postoperative period, and each required reoperation for repair of the cuff tears. Two patients had displacement of their high-density polyethylene components, one associated with a severe traumatic episode and posterior shoulder dislocation, and the second associated with recurrent posterior subluxation and eventual plastic deformation of the polyethylene and its separation from the metal base.

An encouraging part of this continuing evaluation is the absence of glenoid loosening and the almost complete absence of lucent lines around the glenoid. Only one of the patients with the cemented glenoid component has developed a lucent line, and this is less than 1 mm thick and incomplete. No patients in the uncemented group exhibit any lucencies.

At this stage we may conclude that the early results seem equivalent to the early results of cemented implants, and that adequate primary fixation of the glenoid component to the scapula is possible. It remains uncertain at present whether or not the fixation of the ingrowth components will become permanent and will lessen the need for revision of total shoulder arthroplasties. Realistically, it will probably be at least five years before this question can be answered with any degree of certainty.

## Discussion

*Chairman:* Do you require a certain minimum of bone stock in the glenoid for attachment of the implant?

*Cofield:* At present this implant is still undergoing clinical trials, and I use it only in patients with solid bone. I would not use it in patients with moderate or severe osteoporosis. I would go ahead and use it in an osteoarthritic patient with a localized bone defect that could be augmented by bone grafting. So there are limitations. In my experience, use of the implant is most seriously limited by the fact that it comes in only one size.

# Reconstruction of the Glenoid in Total Shoulder Arthroplasty

P. Welsh, D. Gazielly, G. Bousquet

One of the problems that continues to confront the surgeon faced with major shoulder reconstruction is the relatively poor support offered for any implant by the paucity of bone substance in the scapula. The glenoid is at best a shallow dish, and this is often further eroded by disease, causing a breakdown of marginal support which compounds the difficulties of reconstruction. As if this were not enough, the neck of the scapula is flimsy and fragile with a small, narrow cancellous cavity and a cortical shell that is easily perforated.

Many implants have been devised for the shoulder in an effort to reconstitute the articulation. Some are constrained, others unconstrained, and still others semiconstrained in that a subacromial spacer is used to substitute for deficient cuff function.

Current trends in total shoulder arthroplasty favor a resurfacing type of procedure in which the glenoid is reconstructed with bone grafts if necessary, and the glenoid component is secured with polymethylmethacrylate cement. Such techniques necessitate excavation of the cancellous bone from the glenoid and, after careful preparation, the introduction of cement. While reports of glenoid loosening are infrequent in the short term, lucent lines are commonly seen between the cement and bone, and it is likely that further deterioration will become apparent with passage of time, in the same manner that acetabular loosening has become a late problem in total hip replacements. This is cause for concern, because the destruction of the supporting bone leaves little if any potential for reconstructive salvage later on. These considerations led us to seek alternative approaches to glenoid fixation in the hope that we could improve it without jeopardizing the possibility of later salvage should failure occur.

Dr. Gilles Bousquet of St. Etienne, France, successfully used a ceramic-coated anchoring screw in hip reconstruction and in patellar resurfacing. It was felt that the cancellous cavity of the glenoid offered an opportunity for applying this anchoring technique. The system employs a ceramic-coated screw with a hollow central core into which a conical pin is impacted (Fig. 1). This pin bears the polyethylene resurfacing component, which interfaces with a standard humeral component of the Neer type (Fig. 2).

If the screw core can be centrally placed in the neck of the scapula, this technique would appear to be ideal for prosthetic resurfacing of the glenoid. Before the screw core is inserted, preliminary shaping of the glenoid cavity is necessary to ensure that the polyethylene face will be properly oriented. Once the correct alignment has been established, the central peg of the polyethylene component is impacted into the screw core.

At present this system is only in the developmental stage regarding its application in the shoulder. But basic research work in animals by Dr. Gazielly and Dr. Bousquet has shown that the material is excellently tolerated by the bone, and that the implant becomes closely invested by bone within three months of implantation. Given the great success that has been achieved in hip arthroplasty with an unce-

Shoulder Replacement
Eds.: Kölbel/Helbig/Blauth

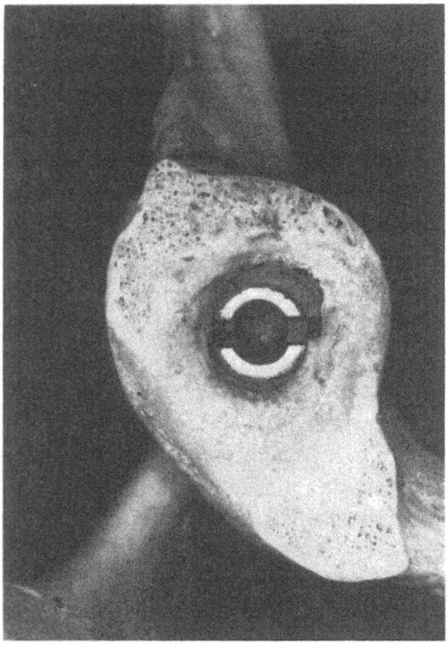

**Fig. 1.** Ceramic-coated screw core inserted in the glenoid

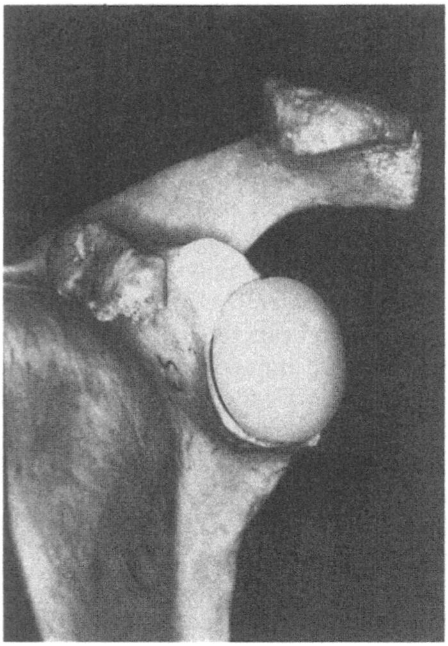

**Fig. 2.** Polyethylene resurfacing component for the glenoid

mented system of this type, it is reasonable to expect that the system will have excellent long-term stability.

Further development is still needed, especially with regard to standardizing the procedure and simplifying the placement of the central core so that alignment of the polyethylene face will be absolutely correct. However, preliminary work on this system has been highly favorable, and we intend to pursue this attempt to use a cementless form of fixation for attachment of the glenoid component.

## Discussion

*Chairman:* As your project continues, do you plan to test the anchorage of the glenoid component for strength? What forces would you use to stress the implant and the fixation?

*Welsh:* Yes, we are in the process of preparing such tests. The test apparatus was designed by a company in Lyon. Load tests have already been done on the mounting knob of the patellar prosthesis, and we want to perform similar tests for the shoulder.

*Marquardt:* If the anchoring peg conical or cylindrical?

*Welsh:* Conical.

# Author Index

# Subject Index

MIX
Papier aus verantwortungsvollen Quellen
Paper from responsible sources
FSC® C105338

If you have any concerns about our products,
you can contact us on
**ProductSafety@springernature.com**

In case Publisher is established outside the EU,
the EU authorized representative is:
**Springer Nature Customer Service Center GmbH**
**Europaplatz 3, 69115 Heidelberg, Germany**

Printed by Libri Plureos GmbH
in Hamburg, Germany